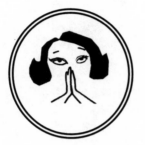

BEEN THERE, HAVEN'T DONE THAT

BEEN THERE, HAVEN'T DONE THAT

A VIRGIN'S MEMOIR

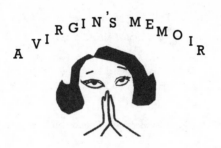

BY TARA McCARTHY

WARNER BOOKS

A Time Warner Company

The stories here are true and unchanged. The names of individuals in this book
have been altered to protect their privacy.

Warner Books, Inc., 1271 Avenue of the Americas, New York, NY 10020

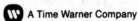 A Time Warner Company

Printed in the United States of America
First Printing: June 1997
10 9 8 7 6 5 4 3 2 1

Library of Congress Cataloging-in-Publication Data

McCarthy, Tara.
    Been there, haven't done that : a virgin's memoir / Tara McCarthy.
        p. cm.
    ISBN 0-446-52084-5
    1. Young women—Sexual behavior—Case studies.   2. Virginity—Case
studies.   3. McCarthy, Tara.   I. Title.
HQ27.5.M323   1997
306.7'0835'2—dc20   96-34404
                                                          CIP

Book design and composition by L&G McRee

For my mother

Acknowledgments

First and foremost, I would like to thank the "characters" who fill this book—friends, acquaintances, boyfriends, and those we'll refer to as gentleman callers—because without them I wouldn't have had a story to tell. Without exception (well, maybe one or two) they are better people than the glimpses of them given here may lead readers to believe; matters of the heart often distort things. To all of them—and you know who you are—I'd like to say that if I've ruffled any of your feathers, it was only in the spirit of telling a story I thought might be of some benefit to others.

I'm especially grateful to my editor, Rick Wolff at Warner Books, for treating me like a writer first and a virgin second, and to my agent, Daniel Greenberg at James Levine Communications, for being more attentive to my work—and more attentive to *me*—than I ever imagined an agent would or could be. I'd also like to thank Verlyn Klinkenborg, who unwittingly put me on the road to writing this book back in college.

Deepest thanks to my brother, godmother, family, and friends (including but not limited to Steve, Colleen, Lorraine, and Melissa) for not thinking I was crazy for going ahead with this. And last but definitely not least, I'm eternally grateful for and to my father; he has been unfaltering in his support in spite of the fact that he now knows much more about his daughter than any father should ever have to.

"My own belief is that there is hardly anyone whose sexual life, if it were broadcast, would not fill the world at large with surprise and horror."

—W. SOMERSET MAUGHAM

iNTRODuCTioN
Kevin Parks

From here on, I'll call him just plain old "Kevin," but it's important that you understand he never attained actual first-name status in my life. None of my friends ever met him. I never really talked about him, and if I did he was always "my friend Kevin . . . Kevin Parks . . . the one I met last summer." Any number of roommates I had during the time I knew him found themselves taking phone messages from him, only to ask later, "So who's Kevin Parks?"

Maybe you're a bit curious, too.

I met him in New York the summer between my junior and senior years of college, when I was living in the Village and interning at *Spin* magazine. An aspiring rock journalist, I went to the New Music Seminar—a week-long music industry powwow—believing it would do my career no end of good. There, I noticed Kevin because he met my three requirements in men at the time: he was tall, he was cute, and he wore Doc Martens. I finally got up the courage to introduce myself during one of the seminar's nightly band showcases and it turned out that Kevin, too, was an aspiring rock hack. We talked for a while, mostly about music and the seminar, and got along pretty well, exchanging phone numbers and a promise to get together soon.

When we did, and Kevin asked me whether I had a boyfriend, which I didn't, he said, "Well, hey!" offering his services politely. But it would be months before anything came of our flirtation, and then only after much alcohol had been consumed.

I was home from college for Christmas and my plans with some friends fell through. I called Kevin, and it just so happened that his friends had copped out on him, too. We went out for Indian food and talked about the pathetic state of our respective love lives, then went to a bar where we paid ten dollars to drink all we wanted and got more than our money's worth.

Back at Kevin's place, sitting on the couch and guzzling water optimistically, we discussed the pros and cons of a one-time hookup. We were both "adults." We both wanted it. There would be no strings attached, and no one would ever have to know. (Until now, I guess.) The couch was soon abandoned in favor of the bed, and what started out as a clumsy teeth-clashing session escalated into full-blown fooling around. We were both pretty near naked by the time Kevin stopped and pulled away.

"There's something I need to tell you."

He said it very somberly, and paused before continuing.

"I'm a virgin."

"Don't worry about it," I said, inwardly surprised to be on the receiving end of such a confession. "So am I."

"You *are?!*" he asked, stunned. Then, rolling back on top of me to resume our activities, "You don't act like it."

To this day I'm not sure what I was supposed to be doing differently. Should I have been pretending that I wasn't enjoying myself? Giggling whenever he tried to touch me and saying "What's that?" when I felt his erection pressed against me? Should I have been writhing around in a white dress singing "Like a Virgin"?

I always hated that Madonna song. The *"touched for the very first time"* bit, in particular. I've been touched, kissed, poked, prodded, rubbed, caressed, sucked, licked, bitten—you name it.

More times than I'd like to admit.

Perhaps I should explain . . .

I'm 25 years old and I'm a virgin. At least by popular standards.

I've never had sexual intercourse.

I am not a right-wing religious fanatic nor am I a

prude. I'm not a wallflower nor have I ever had any trouble finding guys who would sleep with me. I've actually shared beds with quite a few.

It could be argued that I'm a nerd, I'll admit. I always did well in school and graduated from an Ivy League college with a relatively high GPA four years ago. But I am most definitely not a geek. I have a lot of friends, I always have, and I could say that I'm attractive without having to sue myself for libel. I'm probably what you call well adjusted, in that I like to go out drinking with my friends pretty often, but I also hold down a steady job, make my bed on most days, and understand the difference between reality and entertainment. I go to movies. I go to clubs and concerts. I'm more than functional at social activities like dancing, ice skating, skiing, and bowling, and I discovered just last night that I have a knack for those basketball frenzy games you often see in bars. I have good days and bad days at pool. I buy a lot of CDs. I have a life.

The decision to have a life without premarital sex playing a part in it is not an easy one to make. Still, it's one that I made a very long time ago and have stuck to with surprisingly few regrets. It would be easy to say that I decided to wait because of AIDS; not having sex because you fear for your life is somehow easier for people to understand. But my decision was made before I'd even heard of AIDS, before I'd ever even kissed a guy, so potential HIV infection was never a deterrent.

Maybe my decision was made *for* me to an extent when my mother stood at our kitchen sink peeling a cucumber, of all things, and told 10-year-old me that sex is something that two people who really love each other do together.

It's a decision that has been reaffirmed many times when a guy I'm with wants to go all the way and a voice inside me asks *Is he the one?* Sometimes I want to answer back, *Yes, this is the one. This is the one I've been waiting for.* But I haven't yet had the good fortune of finding the man of my dreams or even been lovestruck enough to believe that I have for very long.

Sometimes the question is different: *Will this mean nearly as much to him as it does to me?* And there the answer has almost always been a resounding one: *Not a chance.*

For a couple of years, as my friends began to lose their virginity, I had a woe-is-me attitude toward my own unpenetrated state. *Why can't I just fall in love with someone who falls in love back, have sex, and live happily ever after? Why can't I just do it with the next guy I happen to hook up with, giving into physical desire without so much as a second thought? Why can't I acquire the "just get it over with" mentality so many other people seem to have?*

For years I waited with great anticipation for my attitude toward sex to change. I knew that Catholic girls were supposed to go nuts when they got to college. Alas, four years away at school passed without any change in my sexual status. Then after college I moved to Dublin, landed a job at a music magazine, and felt like I was truly living my own life for the first time ever. I took up smoking. I frequented pubs and rock clubs. I rolled joints with soundmen in Belfast and spent nights with long-haired lead singers and spiky-haired synthesizer players. I'd managed the drugs and enough rock 'n' roll to make up for the fact that the drug was only hash. It only made sense that sex would follow. What could possibly stop me now?

It took the abrupt end of a serious, year-long intercourse-free relationship with a man I loved to finally make me admit the depth of my commitment to saving sex for marriage. To make a long story short, he stopped calling. Two thoughts were left jockeying for prominence in my mind: *What a fucking wimp*, and *Thank God I didn't have sex with him*. Would I really have wanted to give myself completely to someone who couldn't even tell me to my face that we were through after claiming I was the woman of his dreams for over a year?

After twenty-five years, you would think I'd be in a hurry. Truth is, I've had very satisfying, very intimate physical and emotional relationships with men in my life. I honestly do not feel like I'm missing out on anything except the elation I've seen women feel when a late period finally arrives. ("Spoken like a true virgin," one male friend noted.) After being burned by someone I really trusted, I'm more convinced than ever that sex is not something to rush into.

These days everyone seems to look at young people in America, toss them a condom, and say, "Well, they're going to do it anyway." It's true. They are. I hope to God that someday I will, too.

I guess I'm here to say that it doesn't have to be tomorrow or next year . . . or even the year after that.

This is my story.

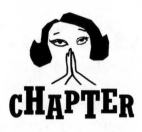

cHaptEr

1

They say that you have to kiss a lot of frogs to find a prince and I am living proof.

For a while I actually kept a list of guys I kissed on the back page of my journal. I updated it religiously for a couple of years, but once I started having to use last names to differentiate the Chris's, Tim's, and Matt's of the lot, I gave up. There was suddenly a disturbing number of cases in which I had no idea what those last names were.

Every once in a while I still think it might be fun to try to come up with a complete list, but it may have reached the point where there are more kisses I'd prefer to forget than remember. Besides, after ten years of smooching, such a list could probably rival a small-town phone book and I'm not sure this is something I'm proud of. For these reasons, you will not read about them all here.

Suffice it to say that number one—and I emphasize that this is strictly in a chronological sense—was Harry Taylor. His name, like others here, has been changed to spare him some embarrassment, but trust me when I say that the name "Harry" captures his glamour all the same.

This was back in the days when you were usually "going out" with someone before you did anything with them. They'd actually have to ask you, "Will you go out with me?" and you'd have the option to choose. The answer was usually a practiced yes, because by the time the question got around to being asked, your people had talked to his people and told them that if he was interested, well, then you might be interested, too. It was, I'm convinced, a question that was never asked cold.

A lot of the times you didn't actually *go* anywhere when you were going out with someone, since neither of you was old enough to drive. It was understood that if someone asked you, "Will you go out with me?" he meant it in a general way—not as an invitation to the movies that night.

This was back when we called kissing someone "going with" them. "Did you go with him?" your friends would ask after you and the guy of your choice came back from a walk at a party. And if you were cool, you knew better than to reply, "Go where?"

So Harry and I were going out with each other before we went with each other, if you follow. We'd met in the

Bishop Malloy High School marching band. Harry was a junior at Malloy, a boys' school, and I was a sophomore at one of its sister schools, St. Stephen's Girls Academy. Stephen's was one of a handful of girls' schools that supplied the flag twirlers in the band's color guard. The band was every member's life for a solid four months out of the year—during which we competed with other bands in the northeast—with the commitment ebbing a bit in the off-season. It was responsible for our social lives, however, year-round. The Dillon family Halloween bash—Jay, Kelly, and Eddy were all in the band—was a particularly notable social event on the band calendar each year.

This year, Harry and I looked forward to the Dillon party as an opportunity to get to know each other a little better. It fell on the same night that clocks were to be set back for Eastern Standard Time and we had every intention of making good use of that extra hour. We ended up sitting against this large rock on a useless little plot of land around the corner from the Dillons' house. I remember being confused about what was going on inside my mouth and saying we should head back to the party when I felt his hand touch actual flesh on my lower back.

Another night, after seeing a Freddy movie with friends of Harry's, we found ourselves on one of Staten Island's beaches in the company of rocks once again. I know we're talking Staten Island, home of the world's largest garbage dump, and not Cancún, but I'd always believed beaches to be wonderfully romantic places. This night, the combination of a startlingly clear sky, invigorating autumnal gusts, and the rhythmic lapping of waves played into my romantic fantasy. Harry's tongue, on the other hand, did its best to kill the mood.

I swear it must have been the longest tongue known to man; unfortunately at the time I was innocent of the ways in which such a tongue could give pleasure and for all I know Harry was, too. When lips locked it seemed as though we were playground enemies who were sticking our tongues out at one another without realizing how close we were standing.

Our kisses were only one of several indications that we were not meant to be. My brother Sean, for one, thought Harry was a complete sleaze and played the protective older brother for the first time in his life, expressing stern disapproval. He was under the impression that Harry was "fast" and that I'd be taken advantage of and marked for life. Unlike Hester Prynne's scarlet *A* for adulteress, the letter we feared was the dreaded *S*.

As in slut.

Only I wasn't so easily seduced. After a month or so my interests were already wandering. Whereas Harry was one of those classic rock types—a fan of The Who, Led Zeppelin, The Doors, and the Stones—David McCormick, my next romantic interest, was more my speed with interests that delved into punk and New Wave. He had short, classic hair to Harry's unkempt, overgrown curls, and cool button-down shirts to Harry's faded Deep Purple T's. Then, of course, there was the simple fact that David's name was, well, not Harry. By all appearances he was more my type and my brother was no doubt pleased with my change of fancy.

I met him on the Staten Island Rapid Transit, a system that consists solely of one train route. It runs from St. George, where it connects with the Staten Island Ferry to form a hellish if popular commute to Manhattan, to the far side of the island—relatively rural residential areas called the "South Shore" or "boondocks" depending on whom you ask.

For me and my friends, the 2:40 train home from school was a point of obsession. Catching "the 2:40" meant a chance to ride with the Malloy guys heading toward the boondocks. The 3:00 train, the other option, boasted dumb macho guys and big-haired, bitchy girls from St. John's who would fake farts and make fun of our uniforms, respectively. Saddle shoe season on the Stephen's uniform calendar would elicit a witty "Going bowling?" every year without fail. Most years more than once.

The only problem with the 2:40 was that St. Stephen's Academy let out at 2:29 every day and the trip from school to the train station was, realistically, fifteen minutes. But the best things in life are worth fighting for . . .

At lunch time we would meticulously pack our book bags and set our combination locks for easy opening. At day's end we'd walk calmly past Sister Octavia's post at the end of the hall, saying "See you tomorrow, sister" without letting on that we were already winded from the run between our last class and our lockers. We cursed green lights that failed to keep the buses within reach for that extra ten seconds we needed to cross the street, and often darted across four lanes of traffic with all the naiveté of deer. I once slammed into the side of a car on the bridge over the tracks as the 2:40 pulled into the station, leaving its concerned driver baffled as I went on to catch the train, shouting "Sorry!" over my shoulder in case I'd made a dent.

One particularly traumatic afternoon, Sister Alexander, my math teacher of four years and one of the most fear-inspiring nuns to ever walk the earth, saw my speed-walk down the hill break into a run. The #7 bus was pulling up at the stop at the school's gate and I absolutely *had* to catch it to make the 2:40. Sister Alexander summoned me inside from her open window.

"What's your hurry, missy?" she asked, as if she would understand if I told her.

"My piano lesson, sister," I lied.

She would release me in time to catch the 3:00 full of shattered dreams. See, David McCormick rode the 2:40. He lived even farther into "farmland" than I did, so each train ride provided a solid twenty minutes of contact. Fortunately, it also provided a good ten minutes' preparation time from when we got on to when the boys joined us. Since you never knew who'd be on the train on any given day, you had to be ready for action at all times. We'd hike up our skirts and whip out blush, eyeliner, and lip gloss from the hidden recesses of our book bags, applying them hurriedly whenever the train made a stop.

Makeup was a no-no at Stephen's and on occasion, evil SIRT riders—perhaps alumnae who'd actually played by the rules—would call up the principal and report our illegal makeovers. Sister Gertrude would berate those people disrespecting the school uniform—"You know who you are"—over the P.A. the morning after receiving such a call, but never made a particularly big deal of it; I think even she knew that a bit of hair spray and blusher could hardly transform us into sexpots when working against the overwhelming dulling effect of our blue-gray polyester uniforms.

Speaking of dull, David, it turned out, was not the most exciting or motivated of people. He had neither the inclination to go out to movies, for example, nor the allowance or part-time job to provide the cash flow to do so. For lack of anything else to do under the circumstances, I used to go over to his house a lot. My mom worried that David's parents weren't always home when I visited (they weren't) and wanted to know exactly what it was that my latest beau and I did together.

I'm not sure how David and I wasted away so many hours, but it wasn't by doing what Mom most feared. David's best friend Robert lived in a house right behind his and they used to play commando-type games, snort spices, and otherwise mutilate themselves. I suppose I used to watch. The two of them were inseparable to the point of annoyance, and I eventually took to calling them "Davert" or "Robid," depending on which one of them walked into the room first. In the rare moments when

David and I *were* alone, we'd kiss, but it never went any further than that. More important, the kisses we shared were about as erotic as a cookie abandoned by a slobbering toddler; I imagine that if my mom had had a chance to sample David's technique she would have slept much more soundly.

I truly believe this was the kind of stuff that kept my mother up at night. She'd lived a simpler life than I would, in many ways, having met my father in high school (She'd gone to Stephen's!) and gotten engaged as a junior in college. When she got married in a textbook Catholic ceremony a few months after graduating, there was no question she'd wear white and mean it.

An elementary school teacher who was home every day by four and all the time during summers, my mother was a real "mom," the kind who made meatloaf, did needlepoint, even made Christmas ornaments out of sequins, pins, ribbons, and Styrofoam balls for the school fair. She was active in any organization relating to my brother and me that she could get her hands on (president of the Band Parents Association and whatnot) and could pull together a fund-raising event as easily as she could a simple dinner for four. When we were little, and other kids were shipped off to summer camp, Mom helped my brother and me and the remaining neighborhood kids set up lemonade stands, organize clubhouses, put on shows, or go on treasure hunts in the woods across the street. She was so clever and creative in her parenting you would have thought she'd studied it in college, and I guess in a way she had.

My father was the sterner, more mysterious parent, or at least he seemed that way to me when I was little. Catholic wedding to the contrary, he was the family pagan of sorts, accompanying us to mass on Easter and Christmas only when Mom's persuasive powers were at her best. The idea of struggling with your faith probably took on a whole new meaning for Mom, who had to coerce Sean and me into mass each week and go up against Dad a few times a year. Seeing that Dad was generally excused didn't help her case much as far as I was concerned, nor did the fact that Sean was an altar boy and had to contend with the brutal 6:15 A.M. slot once a month.

To confuse matters, we'd come home from mass to find Robert Schuller saying mass on the TV as Dad busied himself with preparations for Sunday dinner. He never seemed to be paying much attention and maybe he really wasn't, but the selection of channel—the fact that it wasn't football or whatever—told me that while Dad might have lost faith in the church (if he ever had any to begin with) he wasn't without a soul. I understood from an early age that faith was personal, unpredictable, and for the most part silent. As a family we never talked about God or whether or why we actually believed in him, nor did we call any undue attention to our religion—not even within our own home. To this day I don't even know how to say Grace.

While Mom handled dinner during the week, Dad usually did the cooking on weekends. True to the stereotypical bringing-home-the-bacon man of the house, he commuted an hour and a half to a job his children didn't understand (insurance underwriting) and packed his quality time with the family into weekends. Dad and I would disco dance in the living room after watching *Dance Fever*, pulling off moves I wouldn't attempt today without collision insurance, while Mom and Sean pretended to be judges. During the week, his arrival home at 6:45 each night was always cause for celebration (At long last dinner!) with Heidi, the half-schnauzer, half-poodle family dog we called a "schnoodle," becoming particularly excitable at the sound of his key in the door. Before he could get his coat off she'd be jumping up at him begging for attention as though she hadn't seen him in years, and I sometimes wondered whether her affection wasn't misdirected. Dad was the one who limited Heidi's domain to the kitchen whereas in his absence the rest of us let her roam about the house freely. He was the one who made her shake with fear, her ears pulled back guiltily, when he caught her curled up in his chair in the off-limits den. Likewise, for me he was the one who frowned on my going to slumber parties or having dinner at a friend's when, presumably, I should be home with my family. But Dad's house rules aside, like Heidi, I adored my father and sought his approval in all things.

In the end, of course, Mom's approval was much more important since she was simply around a lot more. Thankfully, she knew that slumber parties were an all-important part of girlhood and had a way of making

Dad see it that way if only for a few minutes during which she'd tell me to hurry up and RSVP. Mom always seemed to be on my side and I loved her for it.

This didn't mean she wasn't disapproving at times. She was relentless at picking on my posture, correcting my mild case of pigeon-toedness, and nagging me about my diction; she'd enunciate the word *enunciate* ridiculously clearly to make her point. Like every mother and daughter I suppose we clashed most when we went shopping. She'd look at the clothes on the rack—the very clothes I wanted so badly for my back-to-school wardrobe—and shake her head. "Girls your age shouldn't be wearing that kind of thing. It's just not appropriate. Who *are* these people who make these clothes; they're not mothers, that's for sure."

So I had learned the value of modest dress; no skirt too short, no jeans too tight, no neck cut too low—at least not when Mom was paying. That was what my allowance was for, I figured out eventually, and began to save up for my own clothes, little realizing my tastes had already been generally shaped by hers. "Lucky Star"–era Madonna just wasn't me, somehow, and I didn't need Mom to tell me that. She did, however, stress more than once that there were reputations to be had out there, and made having one sound about as pleasant as chicken pox.

In our house, my parents supported the kind of distinction between the sexes that will be familiar to many of you; I was raised with Barbie dolls in flowery pink bedrooms, with chores that included folding laundry, setting the dinner table, and dusting the living room; my brother's model airplanes went with his blue room and chores like taking out the garbage, mowing the lawn, and washing the car. Sean was by no means encouraged to go out and sow his oats, but neither was he warned about getting a reputation. And while there was no doubt that both my brother and I were taught that we could go on to be whatever we wanted in life, I was expected to shave my legs and then cross them like a lady along the way.

Since I excelled in math and science Mom was excited at the prospect of my becoming an engineer. Like many women of her generation, she was a living dichotomy—the kind of woman who wore fur but recycled and wasn't aware that it might be seen as a contradiction—and her argument for my becoming an engineer fell somewhere on the fine line she walked between a traditional and a more feminist viewpoint. I should become an engineer, in spite of its being a male-dominated profession, simply because I was interested in the field and more than capable. In other words, why shouldn't I? The other plus of engineering as Mom saw it was that I'd meet loads of eligible men and would, presumably, marry one of them.

Together my parents made marriage seem so natural, secure, and happy a state that I never imagined myself doing anything but following in their footsteps. I knew there were other options because my mom's parents were divorced when she was barely a toddler. But everyone resented her father so much that his existence was practically erased from family history, and my grandmother, in her shame, never received Communion again. Their split had obviously been a scandal for our family, so that's how I started out viewing divorce. My mom's aunt, kind of a third grandmother to me, had never married, so I was exposed to yet another option. She'd traveled the world and had a successful career, but never encouraged me to choose to remain single the way she had. Over the years she'd press on me that being married was really the best way to be and prayed that both my brother and I would meet nice people to settle down with.

So, from pretty early on the importance of the quest for Mr. Right was something I was well aware of. Of course, I knew there were other things in life to bring happiness and fulfillment—I fell in love with dance at a young age and studied it for years before shifting my attention to the piano, the clarinet, and music in general. I read every Nancy Drew book there was before raiding my brother's Hardy Boys library, and got swept up in the roller-skating craze joyfully via *Xanadu*, but the romance of it all wasn't lost on me. I dreamed myself Nancy Drew, cracking cases open *with* the Hardy boys, dazzling them with my cunning and charm. I longed to be asked on the floor during couples skates and imagined myself catching the eye of the man of my dreams, seated somewhere else in the orchestra, as I played a brilliant solo. I'd go to bed after *The Love Boat* and *Fantasy Island* only to use one of the night's storylines as the basis for my own ship-board/island-bound romance fantasies as I drifted off to sleep, and often imagined myself an Olympic figure skater carrying on a passionate affair with my on-ice partner.

My fantasies were so ridiculously innocent that the word *fantasies* almost doesn't suit. In my mind passion was always at the fore while the heat of passion remained unexplored for a pretty long time. I was captured, simply, by the idea of romance and when I learned about sex in school, there was nothing romantic about it whatsoever. I was in the fifth grade, taking Family Living in the place of Social Studies once a week at my public grammar school, when the biology was explained to me in no uncertain terms. The bit about actual sex wasn't nearly so interesting to me as the idea that I would, some time in the not so distant future, have breasts and armpit hair.

Besides, until you have some experience and some hormones, the world between kissing and having sex is pretty much a mystery. I'd seen people kissing on TV and in movies, and it looked like something I'd like to try. All I really knew of sex, on the other hand, came from cartoonish slides and teachers. *Gonads, penis, testicles* . . . the words didn't exactly intrigue me.

A real vocabulary for sex would develop outside of the classroom over the next couple of years as I conquered intermediate school: *slut, whore, dick, snatch, pussy, cunt, come, blow job,* and the like would pop up in graffiti around school and often be used in variation (e.g., "Suck my dick") in schoolyard fights. By all indications, the people who knew most about sex were the ones who spent their afternoons in detention and summers in summer school.

A nerd by virtue of my excellent performance in school, I simply wasn't one of them. Good thing I never wanted to be.

Yes, there were downsides to being one of the "good kids," an A student who was in the band (gasp!) and liked it. For the good part of a year, I was terrorized—crank calls, threats of bodily injury, the works—by two particularly nasty girls on my block, one of whom had previously been my "best friend" back when having one of those (no more than one) was so important. Mom started blowing whistles into the phone and I started walking home from school to avoid riding the bus with my tormentors, a decision that must have given them great satisfaction. When the timing of events wasn't working in my favor, just as I'd reach Amboy Road, the bus would fly by, with Debbie and Kristen hanging out of their window—always at the back—their heads thrown back in laughter and middle fingers pointing up at me. In bad weather I had no choice but to face them and their taunts, insults that were perhaps unique to Staten Island: "Where'd you get that pocketbook, the garbage dump?"

As graduation from eighth grade neared, and looking back it seems ironic, I'd begun to see my choice to go to Stephen's as an escape. I knew it was the strictest school on the island and that the pressure to perform well academically would be great. But I'd be free of the pressure to be normal, average, or "cool" in order to gain social acceptance, far away from people who thought that forming an *o* with one hand and sticking your other index finger into it was not only clever but rebellious, when in truth they probably couldn't be either if they tried. Stephen's was only on the other side of the island, but its grass was most definitely greener.

Of course, once I got there and found myself a boyfriend at our brother school (remember David?), I realized that the grass was greener somewhere else. Notably Finley Catholic High School.

That's where Ian Haviland went.

He was my friend Carolyn's boyfriend Phil's best friend—got that?—and was so beautiful and so completely hip that when the opportunity to kiss him arose it seemed a sacrilege to refuse. David failed to see my reasoning, but I didn't mind. See, Ian Haviland was *it*.

He was miles ahead of David in the romance department and was as fanatical about Depeche Mode as I was. He wrote me letters almost every day and had them delivered to me through Phil and Carolyn. He came to color guard practice when Phil came to pick up his sister just to see me, and to top it all off he made me a tape—one side mostly Depeche Mode and the other just him talking. He told me—via Memorex—that as a couple we were like a hit single: at first people hear it and say, "What's that, I think I might like it." And the more they hear it the more they like it and the more popular it becomes, and suddenly everyone knows it and it's a big hit.

He was no poet. Regardless, I was more than content with the raspy sound of his voice filling my headphones long after I'd bid my family goodnight. "I thought about you in the shower today," he'd say, and I'd hit rewind and play it again, picturing him in the shower with all the unspecificity of someone who'd never actually seen a guy naked. I found his complete willingness to tell me exactly how crazy he was about me exciting.

The fact that he'd given me concrete evidence of his infatuation made it much harder for me to handle being dumped three weeks later. We lived too far apart and didn't get to see each other enough, and Ian simply couldn't or wouldn't do it anymore. I didn't understand. I wanted to know what happened to our hit record. But Ian was intent on going solo.

I think I was actually bold and foolish enough to try to rekindle the flame with David who, to his credit, laughed in my face. Left alone to nurse my wounds, I found that the love life I'd only so recently discovered offered up its first lengthy dry spell.

I knew I had earned it.

cHAPTER

2

The only thing more depressing than not being in a romantic relationship when you want to be is not having anyone in your life you want to be in a romantic relationship with. Even if the object of your affection is your paperboy or a clerk at your video store, who doesn't pay any attention to you unless you're giving him money, just having someone to think about when you go to bed at night or when you're bored out of your mind at work or school makes life a little brighter. We all have our fallback fantasies—for years I'd use Duran Duran's Simon Le Bon in my imaginary scenarios when there wasn't anyone I actually *knew* to think about—but daydreaming about the rich and famous will get your love life only so far.

So, all across the planet, as the school year or semester or new job starts, as people head off to summer camps and summer vacations, excitement mounts. Because when you've exhausted every other possibility—even your mother's friend's son, who she still insists wasn't responsible for that nasty little episode involving Hawaiian Punch and your favorite white shirt at your thirteenth birthday party when you know otherwise—there's only one thing that can save you.

New blood.

Luckily for me, as someone who already seemed to be exhausting her possibilities at a frightening rate, there was no shortage of donors as my junior year of high school began. Three, count 'em, *three* cute guys my age joined the marching band. As the season began, I had a hunch it would be a winning one in more ways than one.

I would eventually go out with two of the new guys and the third would develop a near-obsessive crush on me. Said crush would cause him unnecessary mortification when a note he wrote to a friend fell into the wrong hands. His fantasies surrounding my Sweet Sixteen party were Xeroxed and circulated for the benefit of anyone who cared enough to read along, and there were more interested parties than either of us would have liked.

As if to keep my feet on the ground, junior year also brought Sister Ramona into the fold as she took over our English classes at Stephen's. She was a large woman whose cheeks were always red, as if despite the love of God she was perpetually pissed off. While she had moments of uncanny good humor, her temperament inspired those of us who knew her best to call her "Rambo."

On one particular memorable day, Sister Ramona was wearing a black dress with two unfortunate buttons falling right where you supposed her nipples were. She stood in front of the class, examining the clothes each of us had donned for a uniform-free "dress day," and fumed. Had she been a cartoon—not much of a stretch with her Blow Pop cheeks and starched movements—there would have been smoke coming out of every orifice.

We were all promiscuous, she claimed. A newspaper article of some sort or another had confirmed it:

EXTRA! EXTRA! READ ALL ABOUT IT!
AMERICAN TEENAGERS ARE THE LOWEST OF THE LOW

She accused us of wearing nothing more than panties and bras under our dresses, as if going without slips was the moral equivalent of military desertion, then proceeded to tell us about a doctor in Brooklyn who was giving $100 to any 17-year-old girl who could medically prove she was still a virgin.

We were all a bit stunned. I mean we'd been given copies of Sister Clementine's Dating Rules—the stuff of legends on Staten Island—and good Catholic girls that we were, we followed them meticulously. We always went out in groups, wore slips in the shower, and never ever sat on a boy's lap without first placing down a book or barrier of some sort.

In truth, and as you can imagine, Sister Clementine's Dating Rules carried about as much weight as a budget travel guide written by Bill Gates, and it was about to become obvious to us that Sister Ramona had done a better job of following her fellow nun's advice than any of us could ever hope to. Standing solidly, hands on her hips, she announced for no apparent reason: "I am sixty-eight years old and I am a virgin!"

I started doing the math: If 17 years earned you $100 dollars, 68 years would get Sister Ramona a pretty decent sound system. . . .

It was one of life's little awkward moments. I knew—or at least presumed—that Sister Ramona had never had sex; the situation here was only really disturbing in that it conjured up images in my mind of what it would have been like if she *had* done it. Sex and Sister Ramona had never shared a brain wave in my head and I would have liked it to stay that way.

I was tempted by her condescending, judgmental tone to stand up and shout that I, too, was a virgin, but at 16 I was too young to collect the $100 and knew that Sister Ramona wouldn't be impressed anyway. She did, in fairness, have a lot of years on me. Besides, admitting to my classmates that I'd never had sex would have been a social death sentence. Looking back, I'm sure no more than a handful of them had done it themselves, but I was at that age where it seemed like everyone was having sex except for me and my friends. At the very least, everyone else did a better job of pretending.

In religion class with Sister Rachel, the subject of premarital sex was always a source of heated debate. If it had been any other nun teaching we all would have condemned fornication and moved on to the next topic, but Sister Rachel didn't quite have the fear thing working for her. She was young—one of the only nuns who hadn't taught my mother some twenty years previous—and ungainly, and it didn't take a genius to pull a fast one on her. We gave her a hard time because we could and I suppose, at the end of the day, doing so made us feel a little better about the crap we took from other nuns; they were effective teachers, there's no denying, and when you really needed them they were there for you, but if we'd brought in an outside consultant the majority of sisters would have easily been found lacking in "people skills."

So Cathleen Fagan, an odd mixture of "rebel" and nerd (she was on the math team but was rumored to smoke), would go head-to-head with Sister Rachel, insisting that what mattered most was the love between two people, not the formality of a wedding ceremony. She was unflappable, Cathleen Fagan, and so utterly unchanging in her opinion that my friends and I were sure she and her boyfriend were swinging from the chandelier every night. Not that we had any idea what chandeliers had to do with anything. (I'm still not sure I do!) In any case, it would take me years to realize that many of the people you assume have been around the block a few times have yet to, shall we say, cross the street.

Andrew Fine, one of the new band members, had been around the block a few times and that was part of his appeal. Compared to the other guys I knew, Andrew seemed downright sophisticated. In retrospect, he was just rich with a well-connected mother. He could woo the women of his choosing with concert tickets and theater seats, and was behind the wheel of a brand-new Mustang before most of us had even registered for driver's ed. A January 3rd birthday was only one of many ways in which Andrew seemed blessed.

Ours began as a whirlwind romance, the likes of which I'd read about in *Seventeen* and *YM* when it still stood for "Young Miss." He asked me out at the end of an after-school band practice and I said yes.

Surprise, surprise.

I arrived home that evening to find that he'd sent me roses, and the card—a simple "Feeling Fine?"—sent my heart aflutter. (Get it? Andrew *Fine*? Feeling *Fine*?) His wit was matched only by his capacity for deceit.

Part of me sensed from the beginning that Andrew was a little too smooth for his own good, not to mention *my* own good. He had all these stories about having dated models, and though they may have been completely fabricated or grossly exaggerated, I was both put off and intimidated by his bragging. Still, I managed to act as though things were going swimmingly. Lord knows I wanted them to be; Andrew had an undeniable magnetism and, maybe more importantly, there were third-row Depeche Mode tickets in the offing.

I remember one particular evening at Andrew's house when he was intent on feeling me up. It doesn't say a lot for my wardrobe that I just retired the mint-green sweater I was wearing that night a few months ago. It had a pocket on the front of it that fell at least four inches lower than Sister Ramona's buttons. Poor positioning aside, Andrew kept acting like he was putting his hand in this completely useless pocket and just happening to come up with a handful of breast (all there is). A week or two later he had gotten his hand under the shirt and sweater and was venturing under my bra. It may have been because we were somewhere where we could have been caught that I didn't want him to unhook it, but I think it had more to do with my sense that he was a slime. I didn't trust Andrew's intentions and the fact that he seemed to be in such a hurry bothered me. After all, didn't we have a long and fruitful life together ahead of us?

I've done "worse" things since then with men whose intentions I've doubted (and, as you'll learn, with Andrew, too). Since then I've learned to doubt my own intentions as well. At the time, however, I had yet to experience physical longing beyond the desire to kiss for hours on end. To be honest, I'm not even sure it had taken on the urgency of actual desire yet. I was curious. The newness of everything I did, and then the newness of doing it with someone else after that, kept me contentedly marking time. Each boyfriend in turn would get his hand to an actual breast with less and less resistance (we girls called it the "slippery slope"), but I was in no particular hurry to get down and dirty with anyone.

As for Andrew's adolescent blue balls, he found help. Her name was Vanessa Wilson. This wouldn't have been a problem if Andrew had dumped me before taking up with her, but he hadn't. It's possible he wanted to have the virgin *and* the "whore," and it would be years before I could play both. Andrew lacked both the patience and the foresight.

His wanderings eventually got back to me and when I confronted him, he told me he loved me and denied everything. I didn't believe him as much as I would have liked to, and Andrew obviously couldn't be bothered trying to convince me. Not a day later the "Dear Jane" letter arrived.

Furious that I'd been dumped in writing by a cheating slime, I retaliated. It's embarrassing how seriously I took the whole thing at the time. So he'd kissed someone else; it wasn't like he was divorcing me for my best friend whom he'd gotten pregnant, leaving me to raise six kids on my own. At the time I thought the capacity to do one implied the capacity for the other, and maybe it does. In either case I didn't like Andrew very much anymore.

More importantly, I'd been mortified. Everyone knew what was going on with Andrew and Vanessa, but no one thought it their place to tell me. The fact that he'd cheated was less devastating than being the last to know.

An impulsive youth, here's how I reacted:

Andrew,

Getting right to the point, I got your letter today. It came more as a relief than anything else because it saved me writing one very similar to it in purpose. The note I gave you the other day [in which I pleaded the case for staying together because I was so desperately in love] was basically written to get you to speak up because it was obvious you were confused or whatever. Most of it was exaggerated and if it sounds mean that it was mostly B.S., it was only because for some stupid reason I wasn't ready to break up with you. When I wrote that I loved you, I meant it about as much as you did when you said it (and I don't think you meant it *at all*).

Today I was told that you went with Vanessa again. Assuming this is true you might say I'm pissed off. I won't even ask you if it's true or not because I wouldn't believe you if you said it wasn't. . . . So 1st I'm mad because you lied and 2nd because I could name 10 people who knew before I did and 3rdly because you weren't even big enough to tell me in a note let alone to my face. My friends didn't want to say anything because they wanted you to be the one to tell me. They thought they were protecting me but were really protecting you, which was a mistake because you don't deserve it.

I have two big regrets about us. First, I should have gone by my first impression, that you couldn't be trusted, and second, that I let you break up with me before I got a chance to break up with you, because if anybody deserves to be dumped here it's you. In your note you said you had a lot of growing up to do—well that's the understatement of the year. . . . I suppose I can't be mad at you forever. You can't be mad at a baby for wetting its diaper, because it doesn't know any better. It's usually forgotten about once the stench clears away. Well, I guess you don't know any better but the stench seems to be lingering. Sooner or later somebody toilet-trains the baby, though. I don't know who's going to do it for you (maybe Vanessa), but if she's got half a brain she'll let you wallow in your own shit until you learn that you can't manipulate people. I'm sorry I had to do this in a letter but nobody's answering your phone. Believe me, I would have much rathered telling you off in person. . . .

From,
Tara

Oh yeah, I really showed him. I showed him exactly how fatally wounded my pride was, how hopelessly infatuated I was with him, and how bad I was at rationalizing my own pathetic behavior in the situation.

As such notes were prone to do in our day, "The Letter" fell into unfriendly hands—those of Don Ridges, a guy who didn't like me very much and may have liked Andrew even less. He read it out loud to an entire homeroom of Malloy guys before Andrew got it so that when he finally did, people around him were cracking jokes about there being a stench in the room.

Andrew and I wouldn't speak for months—in truth, we practically bent over backwards to ignore each other—but would eventually admit how ludicrous the entire situation was. We patched things up and after our senior year, Andrew would start up our correspondence once again with a letter proclaiming that I was the woman of his dreams. After all we'd been through he was now sure that I was "the one."

His girlfriend Rachel wasn't so keen on the idea, but I was. (No doubt as hard for you to believe as it is for me to admit.) Andrew would leave her for me and give me a twisted sense of satisfaction. As if being the "other woman" made up for the time when I'd been the one left behind. As if the fact that he'd left someone for *me* was a guarantee he wouldn't leave *me* for someone else. Not this time.

Within a week or two Andrew and I would up the physical intimacy ante substantially. Within the same time, he'd also decide he'd done the wrong thing and run back to Rachel, whom he controlled as if by remote. Everyone lost a couple of friends in the process.

A year or so later, when that relationship had ended (you knew it would) and before Andrew met the woman who is now his wife, we'd have a final fling. By then, I'd had at least one serious boyfriend and a couple of flings. Whereas Andrew's sexual advances had once been new and somewhat frightening, now they were a matter of course. I would no longer deny that the desire was there and he had never tried to deny it to begin with. We spent an hour in the front seat of his car making up for the mint-green sweater incident.

Andrew would never mistake me for a prude again.

But wait, I'm getting ahead of myself. Back in junior

year of high school, I guess I was a prude—never something I thought I should be embarrassed about when the other option was a slut. Still, I would have preferred being called a slow learner. It wasn't that I didn't want to educate myself in the ways of love. I just wanted to be sure I had the right study partner, and I'll be damned if I wasn't having a hard time finding him.

Tom Evans, whom I'd met through another boyfriend of Carolyn's, was as close as I ever got in high school. For a while—beginning the spring after "The Letter"—Tom and I were a real, established couple. I used to go watch his baseball games. He used to pick me up from Stephen's, parked a block or two away in bold defiance of Stephen's rules against such practices. We exchanged goofy cards and had a favorite make-out spot; "The Wall" was a graffiti-covered concrete barrier at the end of a street that dead-ended at the beach. We had fights and even broke up and got back together once. I went to a few of his family parties, saw U2 with him (David, the wet cookie guy, was in the row behind us), and went to his senior prom. It was the only one of five proms I managed to go to over the course of four years that I attended with someone who was really more than "a friend."

When the opportunity arose we spent hours making out in Tom's basement with U2's *The Joshua Tree* spinning on the turntable. Flipping the LP over (and over and over) was always a chore, but one we grinned and beared. After a few months I had every note of that record and the sequence of songs forever ingrained in my head.

There was a lot of tongue mashing and the occasional hickey. There were strangely endearing moments of battle with bra catches, Tom's eyes squinted in concentration, my body frozen still to aid his cause, and when our activities moved from the couch to the floor and lower bodies were given the chance to intertwine (I always hated the expression "dry hump," but I suppose it's fitting), I experienced my first orgasm in someone else's company.

"Are you okay?" Tom asked.

And I was. But Tom and I wouldn't be for very long.

We were tested in a way no high school sweethearts should be when my mother died. She'd been sick—on and off—for a few years, but I'd managed to maintain enough normalcy in my life that none of my friends realized how serious her cancer was until it killed her. I hadn't realized it much before then. An unsuspecting Tom showed up at my door less than an hour after I'd been told the news and we took off to "The Wall" together. I needed to get out of the house.

Tom had no idea what to say or do and didn't have the good sense to say, "I have no idea what to say or do," which is all I really wanted to hear. He dropped me home in no better shape. Worse off, really, since I knew our demise was now inevitable. A few more months and Tom's starting college would have brought our time together to an end rather gently. I knew the day my mom died that we wouldn't last the summer. What I didn't know was that I was the one who was going to be dumped.

At the wake a few days later, Tom and I were kneeling

at my mother's coffin. He'd expressed concern that I didn't want him to be there and I stressed that I did. He knew I was turning to other friends for support—and finding it—and I felt the need to reassure him that everything would be okay, that he wasn't really as inadequate as we both knew he was at the time. Reluctant to deal with another loss, I asked him to be patient, to give me time to deal with this and not give up on me. I'm sure that if it had been in my mother's power, she would have sat up and said, "Get rid of this dud already!"

Tom's main concern quickly changed from consoling me to figuring out how he was going to dump me for Stacy Lowell, whom he'd met at the wake, without looking like a *complete* asshole. To my mind, he would have had a better chance trying to raise my mother from the dead. Obviously, he did neither and none of the details of the ensuing breakup are really important now. Let's just say that no one involved handled it particularly well.

A few years later, Tom would approach me with an apology and express his regret. Water under the bridge, I said, because, looking back, I saw that losing him was like suffering a scraped knee during a car crash that left me with much more serious injuries to deal with; if I'd scraped my knee on its own, I would have slapped a Band-Aid on it and been done with it. The combination of injuries at the time, however, made me feel things were beyond repair. When faced with an apology years later, I felt differently. After all, he was only a guy.

I still think of Tom whenever I hear a song off *The*

Joshua Tree, and those memories are fond in spite of everything. But it was no accident "I Still Haven't Found What I'm Looking For" had unofficially become "our song."

With or without Tom, I was starting to wonder whether U2 had written it specifically with me in mind.

cHAPTER

3

Who's he?" *my mother had asked, after she first* met Joe Marrano.

"He's *cute*," she'd added almost dreamily.

Then, a question she asked rather flippantly but one that would bug me for years after she'd passed: "Why don't you like *him?*"

We've all been there. It's like waiting on a train platform—schedule in hand, bags packed—for a train that never comes. There's no reason for the delay, at least none you can see—no weather problems, track work, or red signals—and other trains appear to be coming and going as usual. Your train simply doesn't show, and no matter how long you stand there waiting, you're offered no explanation whatsoever, no alternative route to your desired destination: Lovesville, USA.

Joe Marrano *was* cute. He was tall and skinny and had beautiful, big blue eyes. He still does. And I *did* like him. I was just never sure whether I *liked* him liked him. This was the source of our troubles.

While Joe and I didn't technically grow up together, it feels as if we did. Back in the days when there was time to do so, we would talk for hours after school. Life. Love. Death. Faith. Family. You name it. We took any big topic we could grab onto and examined it from every conceivable angle for so many hours the phone company should have put us through college.

Much of our relationship revolved around Joe's being in love with me and my thinking I should be in love back. It often felt as if we'd stepped out of *The Wonder Years*, Joe playing Kevin Arnold to my Winnie Cooper. To this day, memories of our experiences together retain the near-epic quality of adolescence as captured on that show. Everything just seemed so goddamn important. And sometimes I guess it really was.

We were sixteen, and while we were fundamentally similar, Joe and I were at drastically different points on our love lines. He was passionate, stable, and fully capable of really loving someone deeply. I was fickle, flirtatious, and more capable of falling in love with someone's record collection than their innermost soul. This didn't stop me from trying with all my might to fall in love with Joe. Mostly I just fucked up our friendship time and time again because I was so confused. It says more about him than it does me that we're still friends.

Joe moved up to New York from Florida sophomore year and was one of the three guys who joined the marching band as a junior, but we didn't really start to consolidate our friendship until the following summer. My closest friends were too upset about my mom's death themselves to be helpful when it happened. Joe, whom I didn't even know particularly well until he called me when he heard my mom had died, somehow managed to strike a perfect balance between sympathy and a more academic interest in death and dying and how exactly one goes about getting on with one's life. Unlike a lot of people, he didn't have any preconceived notions of how I was supposed to be handling things and, as such, became the only person I could bear to talk to about the whole thing.

It would be foolish to deny that my burgeoning friendship with Joe was a big part of what drove Tom away. And there's no denying that the level on which Joe and I communicated made me realize that my relationship with Tom had no depth whatsoever. Tom himself was convinced Joe would be my next boyfriend, and though I denied it to the high heavens, he wasn't so far off. The second or third time Joe asked me out, I finally said yes.

Though we would "go out" with each other for only about three weeks, that's a misleading figure. Once the romantic question had been posed it would be years before it was really resolved and, I think, years before Joe and I could truly enjoy each other's company again. We behaved much like a couple having difficulty conceiving a child—each of us blaming ourselves for our inadequacies and at the same time resenting the other for theirs. Surely one of us was to blame for our failure to form a more perfect union.

Perhaps it's only fitting that Joe was the first person to ask me whether I'd make love to him. Actually he might be the only person who ever *asked*. Joe and I saw eye-to-eye on the sex thing—we both wanted to save it for someone truly special—and it often seemed like we should be each other's first since it meant so much to both of us. But it was a hypothetical question when he asked it. Kind of like, "Would you, if we were old enough to even consider doing it?" I'm not sure what I said, to be honest. I wasn't old enough—I wasn't even thinking in those terms in spite of the fact that I'd begun to dabble in pleasures of a physical nature; actually having sex was still something I couldn't fathom. Besides, I wasn't in love no matter how much I thought I should be, and that was a requirement the way I saw it.

Still, I remember the day quite vividly, at least I hope I do or Joe will have my head. It was late in the afternoon the fall of senior year when those edgy hours just before dark blended the ominous threat of postponed homework with the secure knowledge that a well-balanced meal was already being prepared for you. I was driving a big blue boat of a Buick, having crashed the Oldsmobile the first time I drove in the rain and had my Cutlass Sierra rights promptly revoked. We'd parked behind the intermediate school I'd attended—I might have even let Joe, who didn't have his license yet, drive a little—and found our way into the playground.

I was sitting with my back to a small red brick building with Joe kneeling or squatting in front of me. We were kissing when he popped the question and at first I misunderstood. I thought he really meant it—that he was expressing a real interest in making love to me—and I was mildly horrified (if it's possible to be such a thing). My lack of comprehension annoyed him slightly; perhaps I'd ruined the moment. Eventually, when I was able to change the subject, we moved over to a cylindrical platform of cement jutting upward from the ground, the useless kind of structure found nowhere else on the planet but playgrounds. I sat on top of it and Joe, who was at first standing in front of me, pushed me back so that I was lying down. As he began to kiss my neck intently, my head dangled over the edge as though I was about to get my hair washed in a salon. It was one of my first experiences with an action or position that seems so dramatic in romantic fantasies or movies, but proves downright silly in reality. I couldn't help but feel ridiculous about the whole thing (the cement driving into my shoulder blades didn't help) and I insisted that I be allowed to sit up. Joe reluctantly complied.

We fought a lot, Joe and I. He grew more and more frustrated with me, trying to unearth a love that just wasn't there and later trying to prove that he'd gotten over me before he really had. And I wondered constantly what was wrong with me that I wasn't falling, that I couldn't accept and return what was no doubt Joe's unconditional love for me. I thought everything would be fine if he'd just lighten up, but that would have been going against his very nature.

Still, in spite of our constant tug of war, there were moments of real beauty in our relationship, moments that made it difficult in some ways for other men to measure up. (A bit sad to use the phrase here when there really is no pun intended.) When I let Joe feel me up—how unjustly crude it sounds when it's Joe doing the feeling—in the backseat of a bus on the way back from a marching band competition, he actually thanked me. Not only did he compliment my endowment, admitting there was more than he imagined there would be from the way I joked about being so flat-chested all the time, but he sincerely believed that it had been an honor to touch them. This may sound strange, even foolish, now. But it was as moving as it was awkward at the time. And in a world where men on the streets see nothing wrong with shouting out "Nice tits" to female passersby, sentiments like Joe's have to be treasured. Everything Joe and I did together *meant* something to him. He truly believed that physical intimacy was a gift, more often than not a gift that a woman gives and that a man strives to be worthy of.

It's possible that it was his attitude toward sex and intimacy that kept drawing me back to Joe. Long after it had been established that we were not compatible as girlfriend and boyfriend, we would spend an afternoon sharing passionate kisses at the beach. The next day Joe's eyes would be filled with fire. He'd demand to know why I did it, when it became clear that for me that afternoon had been an isolated event. Did I think I could just use him whenever I wanted to? We had another encounter in the back of a limo the night of his senior prom. At Six Flags Great Adventure the next day, I was my typically confused, regretful, and cold self. The fact that Joe showed up dressed like an idiot—a John Belushi T-shirt, brightly colored "jams," silly suspenders, and gray socks pulled up to his knees—didn't help. One day I'd think, *Yes, this could work*, and the next it'd be all I could do to be seen with him.

Again and again, my fickle nature got me in trouble with Joe and, as time went on, with my conscience as well. When I look back at the guy I started dating immediately after I called the whole thing off, I can't believe I actually chose him over Joe; we weren't even remotely compatible. The fact that I had no problem jumping from Joe to my newest crush hurt his feelings more than I cared to admit. But I was so infatuated by this new guy for whatever reason that I didn't think I'd done anything wrong. I feel, therefore I act. In the same way, I justified hooking up with Andrew Fine, who was pretty much Joe's best friend, in the wake of his senior-year love letter to me while Joe was in the next room telling my best friend Noel how much he cared for me. Only when Andrew later said that he had only thought he was in love with me because Joe was so in love with me did I realize I'd screwed up. I didn't belong with either one of them and am, to this day, eternally grateful that sex was never involved. It was messy enough as it was, but it was nothing we couldn't get past.

There was never any doubt Joe would be accepted to Harvard. He'd come out of the SAT saying that there were two questions he wasn't sure of, only to score a 1580. When I was accepted (everyone thought I was joking) and Andrew wasn't, there were mixed feelings all around. In some ways I was comforted that Joe would be there. In others, I was desperate to escape what sometimes felt like a critical eye; Joe wanted the best for me and never thought my taste in men indicated that I wanted it for myself. We would grow apart socially at Harvard, but we still had our share of traumas, one of which came about when Joe's sophomore-year roommate James and I (we'd taken French together) developed an interest in one another. All of that aside, Joe and I kept tabs on each other, met for dinner when too much time had gone by, and even kept track of one another's sexual status. In some ways we'd come to value each other's virginity as much as our own; there was comfort in knowing that we weren't alone in our desire to wait for the right person, and maybe we still wondered whether in the long run we'd end up being that for each other.

We weren't, it turned out. Joe, who hung on to his virginity 'til the bitter end, found the right person at

Harvard and married her last year. Andrew and his wife drove both James and me to the wedding.

Funny how things have a way of working themselves out if you let them.

cHAPTER

4

We can't say we weren't warned. *It was one of the* first things made perfectly clear to us after we'd settled in at Harvard and we were presumed to be smart enough to grasp the concept: Dating people who live in your freshman entryway. Bad idea.

But we're always the exception to the rule; the "except after *c*" to everyone else's "*i* before *e*." People in the know may warn against things like romance in the workplace or student-teacher liaisons, but, cocky creatures that we are, we're convinced we can handle it. Better yet, we'll *more* than handle it, we'll revel in it—even excel at it. Other people will look at us and say, "Well, *they* did it, why can't I?," only to fail miserably when they try it themselves. Love will conquer all so long as it's our love and nobody else's.

Billy Nolan and I were sure the unwritten rule against intradorm dating was intended for people who weren't as mature as we were. Besides, we thought the pull between us was simply too great to be ignored. So what if he was technically still going out with a girl from home? So what if an on-again-off-again flirtation of mine had ended up in school in Boston and I'd yet to completely sever ties? Circumstances aside and advice to the contrary, we thought dating someone in our dorm made perfect sense. Who better to bond with romantically than someone who'd been there from Harvard Day 1? On top of that, it was downright convenient. Two flights of stairs is a pretty tolerable walk of shame by any standards.

It started with late-night conversations the likes of which none of us felt we'd ever experienced in our lives and maybe we hadn't. The thirty-two residents of the entryway I lived in were downright fascinating to me. During my first week of college, I met my first real-life atheist, my first hardcore vegetarians, people with Asian names I had to learn how to pronounce, a half-Ukrainian black man, a Jew from the south, one half of a set of identical twins, football players who could carry on intelligent conversations. . . . Who could resist such intriguing sorts? Of course, Billy, whom I ended up dating for roughly three months, was an Irish Catholic meat eater with vaguely freckled boyish good looks who might as well have grown up around the corner from me. Though I never would have admitted it at the time, I was probably drawn more to our similar upbringings than anything else. While all the diversity of Harvard was intoxicating, it was scary at the same time. Billy was the proverbial safe port.

Things came to a head on my eighteenth birthday. My on-again-off-again flirtation from home asked me out to dinner, and in the meantime, my three freshman roommates (who ended up being my sophomore, junior, and senior roommates) planned a surprise party back at our two-bedroom suite. Everyone in the entryway was invited, and since we'd been at Harvard only about a month, pretty much everyone came. As freshmen we'd yet to find real social lives so no one had anything better—or simply anything *else*—to do. Maybe it was warm for October or just that the M&M-covered frozen yogurt cake didn't fit in our mini-fridge. It was a mess to serve and I was grateful that roommate Emma spared me the task.

Billy made an appearance that made it clear he'd been drinking—in spite of the difficulties of scoring booze as underaged out-of-towners in Massachusetts— and promptly left in a huff when he saw that my dinner date had yet to make his exit. I think he came back later of his own accord, but it's possible I went downstairs and dragged him back. Somehow we ended up slow-dancing on the cushy pink carpet my roommates and I had pooled resources for. More than anything, I think Billy was holding on to me for support.

We might have actually kissed that night, but since I don't really remember our first tongue-twister at all, I'm not sure. At the very least, I let on that my lingering fling from home wasn't all he was cracked up to be, and Billy said he knew his girlfriend back in Illinois wouldn't last. In any case, I'm presuming lips started locking somewhere along the line, and before we knew it we were seeing each other pretty much every night. We split roast beef heros from Elsie's at 11 P.M., fighting day in and day out over whether to get onions. ("You can pick them off your half," he'd insist, unaware it was his breath I was worried about.) Considering the vigor and regularity with which we chowed away right before bedtime you would have thought we'd been granted immunity from the dreaded freshman fifteen. Looking back, candid photos of double chins serve as proof to the contrary.

Before long we were anxiously anticipating Billy's roommate Rob's frequent weekend trips. He was an outdoorsy type—the call of the mountains luring him and his Birkenstocks away from campus each weekend—and Billy and I were just as glad. It was all very innocent and it's easy to see why. We were fooling around in a bunk bed, for godsakes! And with both of us living in four-person suites, there were roommates lurking around every corner. Under the circumstances, we never even spent a night together. Or at least we never went to sleep and woke up together. Thus the walk of shame at four or five in the morning—clothes disheveled, lips red, eyelids drooping . . . I'd carry my shoes, taking the stairs softly two at a time—*Please, don't let anyone see me*—and sneak into my own top bunk, thanking the people in Housing Assignments for giving me roommates who could sleep through the apocalypse.

I don't know who I was afraid would see me, who exactly it was I thought would peg me as a dirty stay-out. But this college thing still felt like camp to me. Not that I'd ever been to camp, but I suppose that's what made it so thrilling. The idea of a bunch of young people being thrown in together to live away from home seemed like a brilliant hoax some previous generation of youth had played on their parents and somehow managed to institutionalize. For a couple of years before college I'd considered my curfew pretty reasonable. Not having one was simply too much: *You mean I can stay out all night and nobody gives a hoot?* Even if Billy and I never spent a night together, there was a certain level of excitement stemming from the fact that we could.

I guess we just didn't want to badly enough. We were too considerate by nature to hang a necktie on a door-knob and expect a roommate to find somewhere else to sleep in the name of the cause. And even when Rob was away, Billy's bathroom situation was less than ideal. It had no lock and was shared by eight guys, none of whom I was particularly keen on flashing my privates to. I'm sure bolder couples would have faced the logistic challenges head-on—and did—but the opportunity college living provided aside, Billy and I were still Catholic. Not that I saw the inside of a Catholic church more than three times all freshman year, mind you, but you could park the Catholic in you on the streets of Brooklyn with the keys in the ignition and take a trip around the world only to find it in the same spot, completely unharmed, when you got back. Even though we were operating within the confines of a very affectionate, caring relationship, we were sure we were doing something wrong.

In reality we *were* doing something wrong. We were doing a lot of things wrong simply because we'd never done them before. Billy was as inexperienced as I was, so venturing below the belt became part of our routine only after painstaking "I wouldn't mind if you wouldn't mind" discussions. The apprehensive tone in which we each admitted we'd like to be touched between the legs would have made you think we were proposing scatological behavior.

In any case, it was all very innocent and harmless, not to mention clumsy. I became familiar with the feel of a penis if not the sight of one in a strictly lights-off, under-the-covers, clothes-not-quite-removed kind of operation. Activities progressed at a snail's pace, which was perfectly fine for a little old virgin like me. I'd found a kindred spirit.

Then the unthinkable happened. The warnings about intradorm dating started to ring true. "Why didn't you stop by on the way to dinner?"—that kind of thing. The fact that Billy was shorter than me in certain shoes started to really irk me. And with classes in full swing, the urge to find out what else was out there surfaced. Whereas Billy's hand in mine had once made me feel lucky to have someone, it was starting to make me feel like I was back in grade school, reluctantly participating in a hand-holding buddy system on a class trip. *What if the cute guy from Gov*

10 sees me with him? Or that other guy—the one who looks so good in his picture in the freshman registry; I'm sure I caught him looking my way in the dining hall. My eyes were wandering and the rest of me wanted to hitch a ride.

The problem was that Billy knew it would happen this way—that I'd stray—and had told me so again and again. He was a Classics major—one of a few resolute freshmen who insisted they knew their intended major right off the bat—and kept reciting this Greek or Latin quote about women being ever-changing and fickle things. Quite frankly, it pissed me off. And the more predictably fickle Billy insisted I was, the more determined I became to prove him wrong. To be a pillar of strength and commitment at his side.

It wasn't the healthiest of relationships. Nor was the post-Christmas breakup very pretty. For all of his joking about my walking out the door any minute, Billy was devastated when I said I didn't think things were really working. And there was a part of me that wasn't sure I was doing the right thing. I still loved the way he opened his door in one fouled movement, like Kramer in reverse. I loved the way his friends took to calling him "Rippy" (as in Rip Van Winkle) since he spent afternoons sleeping to recover from our late nights and his 8 A.M. Intensive Greek. And his smile was so goddamn sweet. He was a really good guy.

Which was a good part, if not most, of the problem. Who the hell goes away to college to settle down with a nice guy within the first two months? You let your aunt introduce you to "nice guys" when you're 35, single, and craving babies. Eager grandparents ask you about "nice guys" for years—with a you-kids-get-together-yet? glimmer in their eye—because they misunderstood the emphasis that one time five years ago when you introduced them to your *friend*. I'd gone to college to experience new things and ended up with someone who could have been my brother.

So we'd eventually become friends—I'd already gotten pretty good at that—and would work on the same weekly campus paper for the duration of college. I wouldn't say Billy was bitter all that time—I'd be flattering myself—but as he watched me flitting from love interest to new love interest in years to come, the warm midwestern smile I'd once loved turned smug. Almost condescending.

" . . . *varium et mutabile semper femina.*"

Billy figured he'd been right about me all along.

cHAPTER

5

Romantic wanderlust—*that irresistible impulse* to see what else is out there, that resolute belief that someone better is just beyond our horizon—has probably destroyed more viable relationships than Darren Star has acting careers.

No matter where we are in life, we can imagine a better place. Better weather, a bigger apartment, a better job, a bigger bank balance. And no matter who we're with we can conceive of someone else who might somehow be better for us. The fact that no mere mortal can compete with the ideal partners the human imagination is capable of creating matters little when you're the one doing the imagining.

It's the people you leave behind—those people you suddenly can't stand being around—who suffer. They want to know why the fact that they sing off-key suddenly became a big deal, when the truth is it just did. They ask you why you didn't say something sooner if it bothered you so much that they never screw the top on the Coke bottle tight enough, when the harsh reality is that if it were the right person, flat Coke would taste like fine wine. But, of course, there is justice in the world. You dump them and you're free of their bodily quirks and annoying habits; that's what you wanted and you've no right to complain. But start looking for someone else and flat soda and flat singing (or maybe it was the occasional overlong nosehair that did it for you?) are the least of your worries.

All of which is just an elaborate way of saying that if I'd known what else was lurking out there I might have hung on to Billy a bit longer. For while he and I had come as close to a you-show-me-yours-and-I'll-show-you-mine mentality as college kids could get, the guys I encountered in Billy's wake freshman year were more likely to show me theirs and expect me to know what to do with it.

Herman and I met on a ski trip I went on with my roommates when a bunch of people from our bus were hanging out in a hotel room drinking beer. He wasn't classically good-looking, but he was oddly attractive, with dark, deep-set eyes placed unusually close together, an equally deep voice, elegant hands, and a seductively crooked smile. He was more interested in my roommate Catherine that night, but she eventually brushed him off and he asked me out to lunch. We had a pretty good time, but would move on to dinner with less success.

He took me to an expensive out-of-the-way Mexican restaurant in Boston where we starting drinking margaritas and ordered up. The service was kind of slow and by the time the entrees arrived I was having a hard time focusing on Herman. I think I managed to portray a vague sense of sobriety (then again drunk people always do), and in any case was in good enough shape to make it back to Herman's dorm room without having to be carried.

We started kissing. It was okay—nothing particularly special—but all of a sudden Herman was really into it.

"I want you," he declared passionately, as he bit into my neck and fumbled with a button on my shirt, and it was all I could do not to laugh. It just seemed like such a silly, melodramatic thing for him to say. I'd had my share of boyfriends, sure. I'd been whistled at, hey babied, and told I was beautiful by random store attendants, but this was entirely new to me—someone *wanting* me and actually thinking that telling me so was going to better his chances of getting me. I'm sure there'd been guys I was with before who wanted me on some primitive level, but I'm pretty sure none of them had said it to my face. I was used to building up physical intimacy—spending some time on the bases—and the pace at which Herman was heading for home plate was dizzying. The way I saw it, "I want you" translated as, "I want to get laid—bad," in a male-female dictionary and I was wondering whether I'd wasted an evening out with the kind of guy who was going to think he'd wasted his money if he didn't score.

I wasn't feeling too well, having never had either margaritas or authentic Mexican food before, and got up to go to the bathroom. I puked, borrowed a toothbrush, and returned to Herman who had gotten more worked up in my absence. When he made a beeline for my zipper and I stopped him with a firm hand, my wondering ceased.

"You're not ready yet?" he asked.

"No," I said, "and it kind of bothers me that you are."

Herman was miraculously turned off, rolled over, and pretty much ignored me—feigning sleep—until I decided to get up and go. I walked home alone through a major blizzard while birthing a twenty-pound hangover.

I took it all with a grain of salt and was back on the prowl shortly. So I'd stumbled upon a bad apple; surely there were others—good ones—ripe for picking. In fact, I was so filled with the pickup spirit that one night I even managed to persuade my roommates to test their feminine wiles against mine. Before heading off to a party together, we made a bet. Whoever hooked up successfully that night would be entitled to a free dinner at the other three's expense.

The male-to-female ratio was in our favor this night, as it often was at Harvard parties. A bunch of us started dancing and I gravitated toward one of the hosts. His name, I later learned, was Shawn—with a *w*. He was cute, in a goofy kind of way. His eyes were big, his hair curly and messy, and he was a slender six foot three. Combined, these traits made him look like he'd just barely lost the lead in *Big* to Tom Hanks. It was a typically sexual Prince song that inspired him to pull me close and start to grind in a way only Harvard men can.

When the song ended and someone scrambled to find another tune, Shawn offered to give me a tour of the suite, one that concluded, conveniently enough, in his bedroom. After a typical Harvard seduction scene including an extended discussion of Shawn's book collection ("I think Rawls' Theory of Justice is overrated—how about you?") he kissed me. But while I was thinking of my free dinner—I had recovered from Herman and thought I'd make it TexMex—Shawn had other things on his mind. Namely, getting a hand, and something else, in my pants.

I stopped his hand, told him I didn't want to go any further (there I was spoiling the mood again!), and Shawn launched into a lecture about people taking sex too seriously. I mean, it's not like I said to the guy, "I am a virgin, pure as winter's snow and I will not, under any circumstances, allow a man to deflower me until I am wed." I had only resisted his advances and said, "I don't sleep with people on the first date." As far as I was concerned, this wasn't even a date.

"Sex is fun," Shawn assured me before launching into what could have easily been a prepared speech about how too many people have hangups about following their basic instincts.

I don't think I really argued with him. The instinct of which he spoke wasn't really surfacing in me and I guess I didn't want to insult him. There have been a lot of guys whom I have liked enough to kiss. But because there is no middle ground with guys—no breasts—there's a pretty significant leap women have to make from making out to direct contact of some sort or another with a penis. I was pretty new to that kind of contact and simply didn't feel like getting into it here. I'd really been that intimate only with Billy before, and then only after getting to know each other pretty well. In Shawn's case, I wasn't all that interested in what was lurking below the belt, and his lecture did a good job of killing any interest I had in the rest of him.

For whatever reason, he called the next week and invited me out for coffee. For the same reason, I suppose, I accepted. He showed up at my dorm and we made it about thirty yards from the door before he stopped walking and declared, "There's something I need to say."

I didn't get the impression that it was going to be an apology and by this point it wouldn't have made any difference. I told him that he could save his breath, that I didn't really feel like whatever we had was worth pursuing either. No hard feelings. He looked relieved and asked me if I still wanted to go for coffee, but I said there wasn't much point.

I don't even drink coffee with people I like.

I always wonder what kind of women (if any) guys like Herman and Shawn are used to being with. People say there's an overwhelming pressure on men to make sexual advances, even if they're not sure they're ready either, but I don't think that was what was driving them. If it had been, Herman could have easily apologized and taken things more slowly and Shawn would surely have spared me his lecture.

I know there are women out there who go out looking for sex; and I know that I would sometimes be mistaken for one because I behaved too much like one. But I've never been convinced that there are mass quantities of these women (at least not as many as men wish there were), so I can't imagine Herman and Shawn were accustomed to having it handed to them. Perhaps it's simply that when opportunity knocks, most men invite her in and try to screw her.

"There's no such thing as a good man," a cab driver once told me when I assured him that I had a good man in my life, because at the time I thought I did. "Offer them sex and they will take it."

He told me he loves his wife of twenty-five years dearly yet he can't count on his fingers and toes the number of times he's been unfaithful.

"It's not a crime unless you get caught."

Suppose, he argued, that a girl like me decided that she wanted to get laid tonight. It would not be very hard for her to go out on the town and find a man willing to comply. (Truth is, all she would have to do is hail a cab.) But if a man set out to lay his pipe, he'd most likely go to bed frustrated or short a few hundred bucks. Women's power, he concluded, is the power to withhold what men want.

"Not to boast or anything, but I'm probably thousands of times more sexually experienced than you are," he surmised as we stopped in front of my house and I could hardly disagree. "But if it came down to a sexual thing between you and me, you'd have me wrapped around your little finger."

I kind of felt like I already did.

The guy was an asshole, but even an asshole can make a point—namely that men, for the most part, don't say no. If I'd had sex with every man who was willing to do it with me in the last five years, I wouldn't even want to masturbate. I'd be afraid I'd catch something from myself. And because catching something, something deadly, is a reality now, I have a hard time respecting someone who's ready to go all the way with me the first time we're together. I mean, I'm irresistible, I know. But not *that* irresistible. Any guy who's ready to jump into the sack with me has more than likely made the same jump with any number of women before me, and it's downright dangerous to sleep with someone so nondiscriminating.

I once spent an entire party flirting with an acquaintance I'd begun to fancy. He was receptive to my advances and we went back to his room when the party started winding down. Not a minute after we started fooling around, he asked me if I was on the pill. When I said no, he practically cried, "What are we going to dooooo?"

"We're not going to have sex," I said.

It seemed straightforward enough to me, but not to Chris. He looked at me, almost panicked, and asked if I was joking. For me, by going back to his room I was expressing an interest in *him*. I wanted to be alone to get to know him better—and sure, I expected we'd fool around a bit. The fact that Chris just assumed we'd have sex didn't really impress me.

Suppose that I *had* been on the pill and that I was rarin' to go. While Chris's concern about pregnancy was noble enough, he would have gone ahead with the deed once that possibility had been ruled out. Obviously, he didn't have any condoms around or I'm sure he would have suggested using one. Hell, if he'd had a bearskin rug I'm sure it would have done the job well enough for him. Chris had no idea how many people I'd slept with before and no intention of asking. The fact that he would take such a chance on me boggled my mind, and taught me something I was well on my way to figuring out: when it comes to getting laid, a Harvard student, one of the so-called best and brightest, can act as stupid as the next guy. Playing dumb works for some (I'm a poet and I didn't know it), but there's no excuse for *being* dumb when it comes to these things. As a matter of fact, I don't know if I can think of a bigger turn-off. Except maybe body odor.

With *two* strikes against him, Chris didn't stand a chance.

I'd grown curious over the years about what actual sex felt like, but the desperation with which the men I was meeting were trying to get it startled, maybe even frightened, me. Part of the reason I'd never had any real interest in drugs was that I was afraid I'd get hooked, and I was starting to wonder whether sex might have a similar effect on people. Herman, Shawn, and Chris all seemed to be looking for a hit with the urgency of people who couldn't live comfortably without it, and I didn't want to grant anything in my life that power. Not when there was so much else to do.

I knew that men I said no to would simply get what they were looking for somewhere else and the idea that they found me so replaceable, so interchangeable with anyone with the right anatomy really offended me. If it was true, as my cab driver had claimed, that women's power was the power to withhold what men want, I was going to fashion myself a veritable Superwoman. Anybody could get laid, sure. But not just anybody was going to get me. I knew there'd be more men who'd want it—want *me*—and with my convictions reaffirmed, I was ready and waiting.

Ready to tell them no, in no uncertain terms.

And waiting, I suppose, for one who'd understand why.

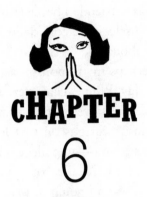

cHaptER

6

My virgin friends were dropping like flies during my sophomore year at Harvard. My Catholic roommate found love and went on the pill. My high school buddies threw Sister Clementine's Dating Rules to the wind and started losing it. I was rapidly on my way to becoming the lone virgin of the St. Stephen's Gang. Suddenly it seemed almost everyone I knew had been lucky in love, and had gone on to get lucky.

I wasn't particularly devastated that my friends were having sex, but the way they tiptoed around the subject would have made you think I'd sold them all chastity belts. I remember Noel asking me for Carolyn's phone number, saying, "There's something I need to talk to her about." I knew Noel was probably contemplating sex and that there was a good chance Carolyn had already taken

71

the plunge, and their secrecy did nothing but make me feel left out and inadequate as a friend. The fact that I wasn't having sex rendered me useless as a confidante and there was nothing I could do about it.

When they did tell me, perhaps my response was not the desired one. Unlike a Judy Blume character who would no doubt have heaved, breathless with anticipation, "What was it like?" I wasn't curious on that level. They'd made a choice to have sex now—in college—and since I was newly recommitted to the idea of waiting until I was married, I figured it was all going to play out differently for me anyway. Their experience simply wouldn't shed any light on how it would eventually happen for me.

This was just the beginning of an awkwardness surrounding the subject of sex that still exists between me and some friends I knew as virgins. It's an awkwardness that I'm not sure exists between me and friends who have been sexually active as long as I've known them. I'm not sure what that means. It could be, simply, that since I'm not having sex I'm not the person friends think to turn to to discuss such matters; you wouldn't, after all, take skydiving lessons from a bungee jumper. It could also be that I overestimate the amount of time they spend talking about sex with other friends or that *I'm* the one who really avoids the subject out of habit, since I did it consciously for a while.

I guess for a long time I'd assumed, by virtue of their being from Catholic homes and their being my friends, that my high school crew all felt as strongly as I did about sex being something to be saved for one person. I think on the one hand I was a bit disappointed in them for "caving," while on the other, I was simply jealous that many of them had truly believed they'd found "the one." What confused me most, however, was the fact that a number of my friends who started having sex were people I would consider more "religious" than me; their faith seemed to play a more active role in their lives than mine ever had. But the fact that they'd made a decision about sex that had nothing to do with their religion—indeed went against it—made me realize that my decision *not* to have sex didn't have to have anything to do with my faith, either. Which was a good thing, because I was beginning to wonder whether I even had any.

One thing's for sure, I was losing faith that I'd ever have another boyfriend. While all my friends were discovering the wonders of intercourse, I was suffering a particularly lengthy dry spell. Perhaps because of said dry spell, I decided to finally reveal in no uncertain terms my longtime crush on an upperclassman I knew. Let's just say the feelings were not mutual.

My mortification was so great, I decided it'd be best to give up on men entirely. My firm belief in the theory that you only find love (or a boyfriend) when you stop looking had caused me to give up men superficially many times before, but this was different.

This time I was serious.

Lo and behold the phone rang and the voice of a

friend at the other end spoke: "There's someone I want you to meet."

His name was Douglas Hartford. He was a junior history major from California who worked as a deejay on campus and was Catholic, tall, cute, and Republican (sorry, but at the time this was deemed a plus). My friend was having dinner with him and a few others in half an hour and wanted me to come along. She was positive we'd hit it off.

Once dinner had ended as far as the rest of the group was concerned, Doug and I lingered over red cafeteria trays. He told me he liked the way I didn't freak out when there was a spider on my tray. It was probably the first time in my life—and the last—that I didn't scream, jump, or at least flinch in the presence of an insect, so at least someone was there to appreciate it. We talked until the dining hall had pretty much cleared, about music, our backgrounds, and why we both felt we should have gone to a more normal college. When we finally decided to leave, Doug asked whether I'd like to come back later to watch a movie with him and his roommates.

As *Slaughter High* reeled through the VCR, the tension began to build. Arms were casually brushing against one another often enough to appear intentional. And as a late arrival pushed his way onto the couch, Doug had no choice but to move a bit closer and stretch his arm out around me. The pretext under which he invited me back to his room was a mere technicality.

"You sure you don't have a boyfriend?" he asked, after he'd kissed me for the first time.

"Yeah, I'm sure," I laughed.

"I can't believe a girl like you doesn't have a boyfriend," he insisted.

"Well, I don't," I assured.

"Well, if you want one, you've got one," he concluded, and we kissed again.

That night, as I stretched out on Doug's bed—fully clothed, for the record—I thought hard about what I was really feeling. He was cute and easy to talk to, but he had the slightest asshole glimmer in his eye. And when that devilish sparkle is there, it's really only a matter of time before it stands up and makes itself known—maybe a matter of weeks before he says he's going to call and doesn't, and another month or so before he finds that a look-but-don't-touch policy toward other women doesn't really suit him all that well. In truth, with so many of my friends coupled off (and coupling), I think I liked the idea of having a boyfriend more than I actually liked Doug himself. That feeling either changed or intensified, and I spent the next nine months going out with him.

No one quite understood how it all happened so fast, but the friend who'd set us up was unbearably proud of herself. Sure, it took a while for Doug and me to get to know one another, but all the while we were doing that, we considered ourselves an item. I guess Doug liked the idea as much as I did.

The day after we met, as I packed to go home for Christmas, Doug kept pestering me for kisses. Or at least it felt like pestering, which was probably an early sign that this was not meant to be. When the subject of sex came up, I warned Doug, who'd already had sex with a few of his previous girlfriends, that it was really important to me and that I had no intention of doing it with him any time soon. He said he didn't mind.

It ended up being by far the most physical—not to mention the longest—relationship I'd had to date. When two of my friends from high school came to visit months later, and we ended up in Doug's room taking a 200-question "Purity Test," they caught themselves asking, "Who'd you do *that* with?" only to realize he was sitting right there.

It was nothing out of the ordinary. I mean I wasn't answering yes to questions about golden showers and orgies, but I don't think the words *oral sex* had ever passed between me and any of my high school friends. To be honest, the whole concept was still pretty new to me. Yeah, I'd heard about "blow jobs" and "going down" on people years ago, but it wasn't something I'd ever imagined *myself* doing. Even when Doug first tried it, I was more in shock than anything. There was definitely an impression in my mind that oral sex was dirty and I wanted no part of such depravity. People like me, I presumed, just didn't *do* that sort of thing.

Then I got to thinking . . .

If this was something Doug—a perfectly normal person so far as I could tell—saw fit to do, well, who was I to stop him? Now that the seed had been planted I was dying to know what it felt like, and if Doug was game, what the hell! Why not go for it? Having rejected his oral advances once before, however, I had a hard time mustering up the guts to tell him I'd seen the light, so the next few times we were together were a bit awkward for me. Doug had apparently given up trying for the time being, and I was so completely preoccupied with the idea of his going down on me that I couldn't otherwise enjoy myself. I suppose after one too many sharp pulls on Doug's head in the direction of my crotch, he caught on.

For whatever reason, the idea of giving him oral sex hadn't been quite as frightening and I was already well on my way to my first blow job, having tested the waters with a few stray licks. After I'd finally bit the bullet, I couldn't find it in me to eat a banana in public for a solid month. The way I saw it, anyone who saw me eating a banana was getting a glimpse of what I looked like blowing someone, and that wasn't something I wanted to show just anybody.

The level of intimacy I'd grown to share with Doug was so far beyond what my friends and I had experienced in high school that they were a little bit surprised; they'd both gone all the way themselves, but perhaps they never imagined that oral sex could stand on its own, that it didn't necessarily go hand-in-hand with intercourse, and that I might see fit to do it. Or perhaps it was just that they were surprised that I'd finally fallen in love.

There can be no doubt I was in love with Doug. When things weren't going well, I could rattle off a fairly lengthy list of everything that was wrong with him, but none of these things really bothered me when the going was good.

Not the fact that he couldn't spell to save his life. Or that he believed California was the whole world and couldn't see himself living anywhere but there after college. Or that he seemed to befriend every fluke of the Harvard Admissions policy on campus; the only interest I ever had in talking to any of Doug's roommates would have been to ask them how the hell they got in.

No, when Doug was by my side and behaving himself, I was as happy as a pig in shit. When the going was good, he'd tell me every day how beautiful I was. He'd come out from behind his deejay table at campus parties and dance with me, and he'd bring me Godiva chocolates for no reason.

It was the *l* word that started the trouble. To my dying day I will be convinced that one night, right before he dozed off, Doug said it: "I love you." So when I decided to return the favor and Doug pretty much freaked, I was understandably baffled. That's about when Doug and I broke up. For the first time.

He'd asked me to go to a campus Valentine's Day Ball and I was desperately looking forward to it. I'd never gone out with anyone who liked to dance and could do it well, so I was really looking forward to a whole evening of dancing with someone I was crazy about. Then my Romeo backed out at the last minute because he got offered a deejay job. I overreacted, dumped him, and went to the dance with someone else.

A few days later, we'd get back together and for a month or two things seemed better than ever. One afternoon after we'd been playing racquetball together, Doug decided he wanted to use the *l* word after all. I was thrilled.

Then, just before spring break I got one of those "I'm just not sure I want to be going out with *any*one right now" speeches; Doug wanted time and space to think. Way to ruin my trip to Daytona. I was sick with worry the entire time, and Catherine and Emma were no doubt fed up with me by the time the week drew to a close. I was convinced Doug was going to break up with me the second we got back to Harvard.

To my surprise, he had a profound if brief revelation (yet another one) while we were apart, and it was all systems go as we headed into the end of the school year. We'd get together almost every night to watch *The Twilight Zone* and Hitchcock and seemed closer than ever. I was also closer than ever to having sex. While there was still something holding me back, something deep inside of me that knew this love of ours was not the healthiest of loves, I was contemplating intercourse seriously for the first time in my life. But as much as I was into Doug, I wasn't convinced he was really in love with me and had no guarantee that this current bliss would last very long. It was as if I knew it would all end in tears—*my* tears—and that if I had sex it'd be harder for me to get over it. When Doug told me one evening that there was this cute girl in his history seminar and he sometimes wondered whether he'd rather be going out with her, I was pretty sure I'd made the right choice.

I think Doug really wanted to be "it" for me but couldn't help himself. He once told me I was the kind of girl he'd want to marry, just not necessarily the kind of girl he wanted to be going out with right now. In other words, he wanted a girlfriend who'd fuck him and a wife who'd waited—the classic double standard. As time went on, he felt increasingly guilty about introducing me to the wonders of oral sex. He felt he'd somehow cheapened me, and that if he didn't end up marrying me, he'd have taken something away from me that it hadn't been his right to take. But for all of his guilt and talk about not minding waiting, Doug was still always trying to get it in there, keeping condoms on hand (and sometimes on something else) "just in case." When I told him that joke about men taking nine months to get out and spending the rest of their lives trying to get back in, he didn't think it was very funny.

I wasn't particularly amused when my clockwork period didn't arrive right after Doug and I split for a second time. Doug's roommates liked me about as much as I liked them, so when it came time for him to find a date for his house formal Doug was in a bit of a bind. He wasn't so keen on bringing me since all of his roommates would be there, so he asked if I'd mind if he brought someone else. I minded.

Crying my eyes out in the wake of this most recent breakup, begging for a cramp or oozing sensation, I was convinced that my life had been touched by irony of Hitchcockian proportions. A pregnant virgin! Now there's a first! (Or a second, depending on where you stand on the matter of Mary.) Not once since menstruation entered my life had a period been late. I'd heard about determined sperm that find their way to an egg, lack of intercourse notwithstanding, and knowing that Doug had come a bit too close for comfort—literally— I figured it would serve me right. Here I was, patting myself on the back for having the good sense to save myself for the man of my dreams . . . it only made sense I'd get pregnant. I'd be depicted as a freak of nature on the cover of the *Weekly World News*

VIRGIN MOM:
EXTRATERRESTRIAL PATERNITY SUIT PENDING

and idolized by man-hating feminists everywhere.

I wasn't pregnant, as you may have guessed, but it took a couple of miserable days until Aunt Dot showed up and relieved my fears. More than anything the whole incident convinced me I'd no intention of marrying Doug. Ever. The thought of having his child had not appealed to me. At all. Still, when he came back begging forgiveness for the formal date incident, I melted. Pathetic, I know. But it was just so easy. I knew this relationship was no good for me, but trying to work things out with Doug just seemed a lot simpler than starting from scratch all over again. He was by no means perfect, but he was as close to Mr. Right as I'd come across so far.

I'd learned my lesson, though, and accepted Doug back into my arms with a relatively hardened heart and a

new sense of nonchalance. I was so sick of feeling inse-
cure that I didn't take the whole thing very seriously. I was
resigned to the fact that he'd surely change his mind again
soon.

Though we didn't survive the summer, Doug would
make a pass at me during the first week of school the following fall. At long last I found it in me to say no.

As the man I loved gave me that look—you know the
look—that "let's forget everything and hop in the sack"
look, I suddenly remembered why I hadn't liked him very
much to begin with.

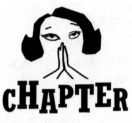

CHAPTER
7

Sometimes, *in the quest for love or romance, we* do things so idiotic that, years later, it's almost impossible to believe we were capable of such stupidity. And even harder still to see what we saw in the object of our affections at the time.

We go on and on at great length, extolling the virtues of our latest romantic interest, only to have to pause, years later, when reminiscing—maybe talking with friends or rereading journals—to make sure we can remember where it was we met them or what color their eyes were. Inevitably, we feel months or years of our lives were wasted—not because the person in question wouldn't give us the time of day (we tend to remember those people much more fondly), but because the person we are now, the person we think we've always been, wouldn't look twice at *them* today. And if we did, we might not even recognize them.

In one of our very own outright dumb adventures, my friend Helen and I got picked up by two guys in a resort club in the Poconos where Helen's family has a vacation home. Or maybe we picked *them* up. These things are never really cut and dry.

It was the summer between sophomore and junior years of college, my breakup with Doug lingering in the air like the smell of freshly cut grass. I'm not sure why Helen and I ended up being the only two people at her vacation house that weekend, but we decided to go out dancing and got all dolled up. All night we did the eye contact thing with these two guys, one of whom eventually came over and asked me to dance. His friend asked the same of Helen.

A few hours later (I think his name was) Craig and I were in his room, while Helen was busy with her new-found partner in the living room. Never mind that these guys could have been psychos, never mind that no one knew where we were (the middle of nowhere), or that we could have been raped; we'd met two cute guys and gone home with them.

We were *that* stupid.

Things were starting to heat up between me and Craig, who had a helluva bachelor's pad and an awesome bed, which is always a bad sign. Virgins, beware beds with coordinated comforters, sheets, and pillowcases! The sum of the width of the bed and the number of dollars he spent making it look so enticing is directly proportional to the number of women who have been or will be in it. (*Minor deductions for futons apply.) Sensing I'd stumbled upon a Casanova of sorts, I figured I'd cut to the chase, never once wondering what I'd do if this guy didn't take no for an answer.

"I don't want to have sex with you tonight," I said. "Just so you know."

"I thought that's what we were doing," Craig replied.

It was actually more of an interesting response than I'd ever gotten. What, after all, is "sex"?

Craig wasn't too interested in pursuing the topic and simply decided to make the best of my hand. As I stroked, he started coaching. Now I'd given hand jobs before and hadn't heard any complaints. And I'd be the first to admit that having someone tell you what they want is a turn-on, but Craig wasn't even giving me a chance. The whole thing suddenly became so orgasm-centric that it wasn't even fun anymore. When it reached the point where he might as well have been jerking himself off, I figured I'd bow out gracefully, admitting his expertise and leaving him to it. I'd always been under the impression that this kind of thing was enhanced by the participation of two parties, but I'm sure Craig had more fun finishing the job himself.

Some would say that makes me a dick tease, the kind of girl that leaves men the whole world over in agony, facing cold bracing showers or bringing themselves to climax. Virgins are always accused of this, as if intercourse were the only way to bring a human male to orgasm, but more interestingly, as if it were written somewhere that upon his birth a man is granted entitlement to an orgasm every time he gets aroused in the presence of a woman. As if the "pain" of an unrelieved erection had been measured and determined to be infinitely more powerful than your average menstrual cramp and more on the level of birthing a child. Give us a break.

Sure, I've left men hanging, but not as a general rule. Likewise, I myself have been left hanging, but I try not to make a habit of it. There have been men I've been with who were so concerned with their pleasure that I didn't feel like providing it. And there have been others whom I've pleasured in numerous ways, again and again, with negligible interest in my own satisfaction. There have been men who've felt it helped to guide my efforts, and others who've praised me to the high heavens, claiming that bedtime activities with me have been more erotic and ultimately more satisfying than intercourse with others.

I don't think the difference between these men is that some are sex-obsessed losers and the others are eligible, marriageable bachelors, though that would be true in some cases. I think it's just that when there's a real mutual interest involved it shows. Over the years, I would have my share of sessions born out of hormones and booze, and they've never been as satisfying—emotionally *or* physically—as connections stemming from a combination of real interest and attraction. But as I took what I'd learned from being with Doug out into the world that summer, I suddenly realized that I had something I'd never been convinced I was capable of: sex appeal.

At the same time, I could finally see why some people don't need to care about the person they're spending the night with—how sex could be just sex, nothing more. I missed Doug, longed for the physical intimacy we shared, and on this particular night in Pennsylvania, I experienced firsthand (hardy-har-har) how fooling around with another guy could serve as a substitute. At the time I didn't want to admit just how poor a substitute.

I would suffer embarrassment and shame in the wake of nights like this one (and there would be more of them, I guarantee you) when the ecstasy was gone and the hangover had set in, but I denied those feelings. And though I was frightened by how far I found myself going in the course of one night—how in the heat of the moment sexual acts can lose any significance they might have had when, for example, you did them the first time—I comforted myself with the fact that it could have been worse; I could have had *sex*.

Which brings us back to the big question—What is sex?—and to the other questions that rush in right behind it. What is virginity? Is intercourse really that different?

A lot of people think that I've come so close I might as well have done it, that my cutoff point is completely arbitrary, and that, therefore, I'm not *really* a virgin. I can't disagree wholeheartedly. The words *chaste* and *pure* often enter into the definition of *virgin* and I'd never claim to be either. I'm probably more in tune with what I like and don't like in bed than a woman who has slept with one or two guys and hasn't ever really fooled around with anyone else. All I know is that I've steered clear of intercourse for reasons that have always been crystal clear to me: it's the only thing that can get you pregnant and I'm not ready to have kids. And since it's the only act that physically joins two people together, in which the parts truly fit, I've imbued it with symbolic meaning and reserved a special place for it in my life. I've allowed myself other physical pleasures for reasons that are equally clear—I'm human, I have sexual impulses and inclinations, and I don't believe there's anything wrong with acting on them. Whether this combination of views makes me a virgin or not, I don't know.

But if you get caught up in semantics you miss my point completely. And that point, so far as I can tell, is that the traditional definition of virginity—one that associates never having had intercourse with being pure and proper—is pretty outdated. And that it's about time.

This whole all or nothing mentality—the virgin or whore complex—has really warped things. There is a whole world between chaste goodnight kisses on the front porch and fucking in the backrooms of seedy clubs, but because everyone's so embarrassed to admit that normal, everyday people like Mom and Dad do more in bed than make babies, it's no surprise that a lot of people growing up today don't realize that exploring their sexuality doesn't have to mean risking pregnancy, disease, and their sense of self.

A boyfriend once said to me that he thought if his parents knew what we did in bed together, they'd probably prefer it if we were just having sex. What's that all about? I don't own handcuffs. I'm not a contortionist. But society shies away from anything that isn't standard missionary-position screwing. There's so much emphasis on the act of intercourse that people aren't given the chance to figure out what else there is—how to be a sexual being without sleeping with anyone with the right body parts. Everyone acts like we're all on this inevitable course toward intercourse—the be-all and end-all—when in truth it's a course you can navigate as you like, with plenty of stops along the way.

I'm not trying to say that the world would be a better place if everyone was going down on everyone else, fingering each other under the table or playing domination games on park benches. But at least, with the emphasis taken off actual sex, two people can enjoy each other's bodies—and their own—with less risk.

As in any aspect of our lives, we make mistakes in our sex lives. Mistakes, if I may echo some bad self-help literature for a moment, are a part of growing up. The best ones to make are ones you can learn from and promptly forget, not ones that you have to put through college.

On top of that there's the fact that if it hasn't already happened to you that you grow embarrassed at ever having had an interest in a certain someone after the fact, it will. You may gaze into your current interest's eyes and swear you see "forever," but give it some time—maybe have your eyes checked—and you'll often find it says "not ever."

At one point during high school I became obsessed with this guy Mike Duffy simply because he was, according to my journal, "Beautiful, that's the only way to describe him." A few days later I thought of a couple of other ways to describe him; "ass" and "low life" jump off the page. Mike and I kissed at a party at his house. The next day, he told me he'd deny we did anything and swore me to secrecy; there were girls he knew who wouldn't take the news of our fling too well. He told me he had friends who could hurt me if I opened my mouth, and since his father was a corrupt politician I believed him. On the way to school on Monday, some of the girls in question gave me a pop quiz.

"Did you hook up with Mike Duffy?" they asked.

"Why don't you ask him?" I replied.

"Well, he says he didn't," they countered.

"So what are you asking me for?" I'd throw out.

Let's just say I'm glad my encounter with Mike never went beyond kissing, heavy breathing, and teenage groping. I enjoyed it in the moment, but had no problem whatsoever moving on with my life. Mike Junior, on the other hand, would not have been so easily forgotten. And if he had a head half the size of his father's, giving birth to him would have been a real bitch.

Back in high school, hooking up with Mike Duffy was probably the dumbest thing I'd ever done. Four years later I was still doing dumb things—like going home with strange men in the Poconos—and I knew full well that there would be more dumb things in my future. There's something liberating about admitting that it's inevitable you're going to fuck up; it takes the pressure off. But beyond that, there's something empowering about knowing that you're not going to fuck yourself or your life up by fucking the wrong person.

There's dumb, and there's dumber, and as I prepared for my junior year in college, I was sure I knew the difference.

cHAPTER

8

There's a reason *Calvin Klein's Obsession is a* success in spite of its annoying, whispered commercials. On some level, it's what we all crave—a mad infatuation, a passionate devotion, a love so insane it blinds us to any of its faults. Never mind that it has the power to transform us into completely pathetic, groveling losers—or worse, evildoers intent on getting what we want, whatever the cost. Never mind our knowing that what really lies between love and madness is a horny person with way too much spare time. We all want to be driven to obsession only to deny we're really there.

I'd seen him before so I couldn't technically claim it was love at first sight. I don't suppose it was actually *love* at all, but at the time it felt like it. In revisionist terms, I'd probably call it "powerful connection at first encounter." Anything to avoid the *o* word.

It was raining that night—the kind of rain you can smell before it arrives. Rain that flips umbrellas inside out (you silly human, you) and makes your socks stain your feet. The kind of rain that actually bounces. So unless you were a resident of Cabot House—like I was—and had the benefit of underground tunnels that linked most of the housing complex, getting to Cabot's annual reggae concert that night was an ordeal.

As members of the House Committee (basically a social committee), Emma and I were collecting money at the door—drip dry—when he rushed in with some friends, jacket hiked up over his head. Drenched. The interchange that ensued was like a strange dream:

EMMA: That'll be five dollars.

HE: Oh, come on, we had to pay for a cab all the way here. How about three?

EMMA: I don't know . . .

ME: Go ahead, Em. He's a Gov major like me.

HE: How'd you know that?

ME: Because I love you.

HE: Great, you wanna dance?

What was I *thinking*? I honestly don't know—except that our first meeting had me convinced that Cadman and I were meant to be. Trying to convince him of that, however, proved difficult.

For me, Cadman was one of those people you care about instinctively, more than circumstances would seem to indicate you *should* care. This instinct does not always mix well with physical attraction. Since both elements were present here, I found myself turning every crumb he threw my way into a veritable smorgasbord, as if the simple fact that I had all these incredibly strong feelings for him meant that he just *had* to reciprocate every last one of them. He'd say, "Let's have lunch," and I'd hear "Let's get married." Well, not exactly, but you get my point. So much of our relationship existed in my head that I could have gone for relationship counseling alone.

He played his part, of course. But to say he read more letters than he wrote and answered more calls than he made (or even returned) is understatement. Years after all the turmoil that you're about to read about occurred, random friends of mine would ask, "What ever happened to that guy . . . what was his name?" They rarely remember such an unusual name, but it's always Cadman they're talking about. If there's one person in my past I babbled to friends about ad nauseam it's him. None of his friends, on the other hand, would have any clue who I am.

My memory of the sequence of events following our first encounter is so blurry it's embarrassing. Fortunately the tale depends very little on actual chronology. Though it dragged on for over two years (obviously with various other relationships occurring along the way), my relationship with Cadman (if it can really be called one) never actually progressed at all. So while it had a beginning and an end—a distinct no-nonsense end—the middle was a big amorphous mass made up mostly of my delusion that Cadman was more interested in me than he was capable of admitting to himself, and his inability to blow me off—no if's, and's, or but's about it—and be done with me once and for all.

First, a confession. The night that I first met Cadman and proclaimed my love, right at the end of sophomore year, I was technically still going out with Doug. I only managed a small kiss before guilt got the better of me, and when I admitted I was seeing someone, Cadman and I agreed it would be best not to go any further. I was still committed enough to Doug that I confessed an edited version of my infidelity to him, but it was hard for me to feel bad since Doug had turned our relationship into such an emotional yo-yo.

I'm not sure I would have been able to put a finger on it—on exactly what drew me to Cadman beyond his being drop-dead gorgeous—before I found out that his mother was battling cancer. By now, my mom had been dead three years and I'd yet to meet anyone who'd been through what I'd been through. At the time—and you may not believe in such things—I figured some divine force had brought us together so that I could help Cadman through it. Looking back I probably needed the help just as badly.

Before the school year ended, and after Doug had already gone home to California, Cadman and I went out together—to a party where we danced and played pool into the wee hours. He invited me to go to the dog races the following day, but lines of communication got crossed (not to mention disconnected) and we never got to say a proper good-bye for the summer. Still, I had his home address and wrote him a letter telling him that he and his family—particularly his mom—were in my prayers and that if he ever needed to talk he knew where he could find me.

It wasn't until the following fall—when I met him at the Au Bon Pain in Harvard Square and he kissed me ever so gently on the forehead—that I found out he had received the letter but didn't really know where to find me at all. Claiming that my letter had arrived at his house with a return address in his home state, Cadman told me he had gone to that address looking for me only to be told no one named Tara lived there. I could never really see how my nun-tested penmanship could be so easily misconstrued, but in any case, I was moved that he'd tried to seek me out and saddened by the news that his mom had died a few weeks earlier.

Cadman made so little effort to contact me or see me in the following months that I had an increasingly hard time picturing him driving through the streets of San Antonio in search of me. But when we *did* get together and talk, I mean *really* talk, we clicked. To this day I'm sure he felt it, too. Maybe he just didn't want to. As time went on, it did start to feel as if the one thing that at first seemed to bring us closest—the shared experience of los-ing a mother—became the thing that drove us apart. The psychoanalyst in me can't help but think that I reminded Cadman of his mother's death and that he was happier to just forget. On the other hand, it's also possible that I simply reminded him too much of Glenn Close in *Fatal*

Attraction. In my quest to soothe what I considered to be Cadman's tortured soul, I sometimes got carried away.

After he and I had lunch one day, we wandered toward Radcliffe Yard, one of the prettiest spots on campus. A courtyard enclosed by red brick buildings and sprinkled with trees and flower beds, it was one of my favorite places to sit and think. A bit off the beaten path, it boasted a certain serenity that the more famous Harvard Yard (where very few people are ever allowed to park a car, for the record) could rival only when blanketed by quiet snow in the dead of night.

I'm not sure how we got onto the subject, but we were lounging on the lawn in the shade of a small tree, talking about all the reasons I hadn't yet had sex and all the reasons Cadman had. I went home that night and wrote a poem (I use the word loosely), and if you promise not to laugh, I'll share it with you now.

> *He stretched out*
> *on the grass,*
> *revealing hairs—*
> *darker than the hair on his head.*
> *And suddenly,*
> *the grass turned to satin—*
> *sheets.*
> *And I wasn't talking*
> *about my virginity,*
> *I was losing it.*

So poetry was never one of my strong points.

Neither was subtlety.

One evening that I'd managed to lure Cadman back to my room, I left a copy of the poem on my desk—not exactly in plain sight, but enough so that a little harmless snooping while I was in the bathroom would unearth it easily enough.

He took the bait.

I think at first he was flattered. Then we were kissing and stuff, and I think he was going to take my shirt off or unzip my jeans or something and he said, "Would you let me?"

So I thought he meant, would I let him take off my shirt or unzip the zipper and said yes. Evidently that's not what he meant at all. Evidently I'd just told him that I'd have sex with him, that I actually wanted my life to mirror my "poetic" fantasies. As if I'd actually do it for the first time with a guy named Cadman . . .

"Do it to me, *Cadman*."

"Faster, *Cadman*."

"Take me, *Cadman*."

Seriously, though, he ripped himself away from me and started pacing around my box of a bedroom like a caged beast. He was just a teensy bit freaked out.

I quickly scrambled to explain the misunderstanding, but the words wouldn't come. "No, I don't mean I'd let you, I mean, not now, maybe at some other point, if things worked out . . . oh, I don't know."

"I think I should go," he said. And so he did.

I'm not exactly sure what it is that's so horrifying about the concept of sleeping with a virgin. Some men, of course, like the idea—even get off on it—and see it as some kind of ego trip. A friend of mine says that the first guy she was with asked her whether she was a virgin right before they did it, and she lied just so that she wouldn't give him the satisfaction. After reading my share of graffiti in men's rooms (don't ask), I can see why. I pity any woman who lost her virginity to the guy—whoever he is—who wrote "You know what's so great about having the biggest dick in the world? It's like fucking a virgin every time" on the wall in his favorite watering hole.

Ego trips aside, generally nice, well-meaning guys don't usually want the responsibility. It's a bit warped, really, when you think about it—this idea that men are taking something away from a virgin by having sex with her, the idea that someone else can feel guilty for engaging in what's supposed to be a mutual act. If I'm responsible for my own body, and my own sexual activities, why should someone else feel responsible for my feelings if they're on the up-and-up? Cadman, for example, had not misled me in any way whatsoever. He'd never promised me anything, and when he did say he'd call or whatever, he failed to live up to his word often enough that I'd have been a fool to believe anything he said. If I'd had sex with him or someone like him, I would have known beforehand that it was going to mean a lot more to me. If I went ahead and did it anyway, any hurt I might have felt afterwards (and you know I would have) would have been my own fault.

I think that deep down most men know that sex isn't just physical. They may wish that it was, and they certainly do a good job of pretending. But tell them you're a virgin and they have a hard time hiding from themselves. "That's a big deal," they'll say. "You want to save that for someone special." They know there's a difference between "sex" and "making love" and don't want to do one if they know you're expecting the other.

By the same token, I think a lot of women deny that sex is more than physical to them and then blame the guy when he doesn't give them the emotional response they're looking for—even though there was never any indication that he would. The solution always seemed simple enough to me: don't sleep with a guy who you think—even for one second—could be pulling a fast one on you, lying to you, telling you he loves you just to get it, or whatever. I had a hard enough time letting go of Cadman; I can't imagine what kind of lunatic I would have been if I'd slept with him, but I'd wager a guess that instead of reading this book you'd be watching a made-for-TV psychothriller movie called *Enter at Your Own Risk*, in which I'd avenge the loss of my precious virginity rather violently.

At 20 or 21, and perhaps because of Cadman's reflex response, I finally realized how much of an exception to the norm I was, and began to understand how that affected the way I looked at everything around me, every man who expressed an interest. It was beginning to feel like my virginity had become an entity unto itself, and I understood that it was one that had the power to make me less attractive in some men's eyes. The fact that I went to Harvard had the same effect in certain situations; a temp agent once told me to take Harvard off my résumé because it would better my chances of getting a summer job as a secretary. I could have lied—spared potential employers the "Harvard," and Cadman, the "virgin"— but what was the point if all it got me was a job I didn't want and a guy who didn't want the real me?

As time went on, my feelings for Cadman became more maternal than anything and I'm not sure the chemistry was really there, anyway. One of the first nights of senior year, after I'd spent a summer writing him innuendo-ridden letters he had no problem sharing with his buddies for the sake of a laugh, we found ourselves fooling around again. It was the first and only time I've ever faked an orgasm, and apparently I've got a lot to learn from Meg Ryan.

"How was it?" he asked, and it seemed like a strange, even egotistical, question.

"Great," I heaved unconvincingly.

"You're lying," he said flatly, and I didn't argue.

Our next encounters were less than ideal. Perhaps the orgasm faking embarrassed him. Or maybe it was the fact that a little while later, I had to shake him and shake him to wake him from a nightmare and stop him from screaming; vulnerability probably didn't suit him. By all appearances he was a big man on campus, someone who had it all together—an A student with an active social life and lengthy list of extracurricular accomplishments to boot. He probably didn't like the fact that I'd glimpsed another side, and asked me to go home in no uncertain terms.

And so it went . . .

I'd run into him on campus and say, "How are you?"

"Late for class," he'd reply.

"Okay." I'd nod, and start to walk away, glad I was wearing a watch.

He'd call after me, "I'd like to talk some time."

"I'd like that too," I'd reply.

Then a few more months would pass.

I'd run into him at a party. He'd be at the keg when I just *happened* to need a refill. He'd begin to fill my cup, and I wouldn't say a word.

"So you're just going to ignore me," he'd ask.

"I'm operating on a speak only when spoken to policy," I'd reply.

Then, inevitably, I'd get deep on him. It was something I did way too often: "I've proved I can be your friend time and time again, but it works both ways and if we're going to be friends I think it's time you prove you're up to it."

He'd nod, almost solemn. "You're absolutely right."

Nothing ever came of any of this, these declarations of intent, and as senior year drew to a close our confrontations got progressively nastier. On the senior booze cruise, I practically formed a human blockade when I saw him coming out of the men's room. He said he couldn't talk, that a friend of his on the first deck had gotten sick, and I badgered him for always having an excuse, despite the wad of toilet paper in his hand.

At the "Last Dance," I found it in me to apologize for the booze cruise thing, and in a rather hostile conversation he told me that he'd never understood what the big deal was. That he'd just fooled around with me a couple of times, that we'd never really been anything more than friends. I said I wasn't sure we'd ever been that at all.

"How about now, then?" he asked. "Friends?"

And he extended a hand . . .

In that split second, it was as if Bono appeared by my side and started feeding me lines from U2's "One": *"Have you come here for forgiveness / Have you come to raise the dead / Have you come here to play Jesus / to the lepers in your head?"*

Of course, I didn't *say* that. I'm not *completely* insane. I just looked him in the eye and shook my head.

No.

Maybe I thought that by refusing to make peace I'd teach him something—and that some other woman in his future might benefit from whatever it was. I guess I hoped that one day he'd realize that I had nothing but the best of intentions, and that some years down the road, maybe when his future wife happened upon some of his old letters and asked who I was, he'd look

back on it all and wish that he'd done a few things differently.

I know I do.

For starters, I would have let Emma charge him five
bucks.

cHAPTER
9

Sometimes you just have to see for yourself—to touch the plate when the waiter warns you that it's hot or dip a few toes into the water when a friend screams that it's *freezing*. This apparent human tendency to want to inflict pain on oneself is so great—particularly in matters of the heart—that I often wonder why shows like *Melrose Place* aren't aired with Public Service warnings: DO NOT TRY THIS AT HOME.

There's no guarantee we'd pay attention, but I think most of us know that none of the goings-on in the *Melrose Place* apartment complex are good for the soul and would have moved out a long time ago. Surely there are other places to live in L.A. Places where you don't have to deal with your ex-husbands, ex-boyfriends, and ex–best friends on a daily basis. Where your lover's ex's aren't lurking around every corner. Where, God forbid, a healthy relationship might make a home.

Most of us know that if one man and his three ex-wives, two of whom are sisters, all showed up at the same party none of them would have any fun whatsoever. We certainly know better than to go to another of our ex-husband's ex-wives for psychiatric help, and the chances of our ever sleeping with our dead husband's brother or marrying the father of our archenemy, who herself is married to our ex-fiancé, are pretty slim. Still, we watch every week for a reason, perhaps the same reason we watch talk shows: in our worlds, in our own ways, we create our very own situations that are just as fucked up.

We fall for people who already have significant others. We start things up with someone only to realize it's that person's roommate or best friend we're thinking about when we go to bed at night. We suddenly find our attention caught by the ex or current love interest of a good friend. And ultimately, despite ourselves, we act on these impulses, entering into secretive liaisons, betraying people we don't even know and some that we do, risking friendships and creating awkwardness for ourselves and others all around. Better still, we're completely capable of rationalizing our behavior even though on some level we know what we're doing is wrong, that in the long run none of this is worth it, that ex-boyfriends of friends are considered off-limits for a reason and that there really is no such thing as "friends who fool around."

For the uninitiated, "friends who fool around" are, as

the term implies, friends. They are not going out, not even seeing each other—nor do they have any particular interest in doing so. At least one of them has made this very clear. This arrangement usually comes about in one of two ways. In the first case, the two parties involved have decided that their relationship—until now a committed, romantic one—is no longer working. At the time of breakup neither partner has anything else lined up so neither of them is particularly interested in giving up a reliable source of orgasm. Disappointed that their relationship is coming to an end, they carve out a compromise and decide that they'll be friends—as opposed to lovers—but that they won't necessarily have to resist the urge to act on the physical attraction that brought them together in the first place. Inevitably, feelings are hurt when one person loses interest completely or the other can't handle the lack of commitment. That being the case, the "friends who fool around" idea does nothing more than make the transition to actual friends, if that happens at all, a more painful and drawn-out process.

In the second situation, two people are drawn to one another but aren't 100 percent into the idea of becoming an item. Perhaps the romantic spark is a bit lacking but compatibility isn't. A friendship has already been established and the fear of losing it is great. But the desire for physical intimacy is also great, and neither partner is getting any anywhere else. At least not as often as they'd like. In this situation, the likelihood of one participant wanting a real romantic commitment but settling for "friends who fool around" is high. Hurt often enters the picture when one partner finds someone who is truly more than a friend and no longer wants to fool around with their friend who fools around. Or when the significant other of one friend who fools around, heretofore otherwise occupied in a state or country far away, comes to visit and the other friend who fools around is relegated to the role of a mere friend. Or, depending on how you look at it, a mere fool.

As you can see, it can get kind of confusing.

When Adam and his friends first moved into Cabot House a year after I did, I had a crush on his roommate Greg. Everybody did. He was that kind of guy. The kind of guy everyone assumed must have a girlfriend "at home" because he did. At least for a while. You could just tell. Nonetheless, being human and possessing that tendency toward the infliction of pain, I had to make it clear I was interested in him before giving up hope. Yes, he had a girlfriend, but maybe if he knew he could have me she wouldn't seem so hot after all.

This was, to my chagrin, not the case. Though Greg and his partner would eventually succumb to the difficulties of long-distance college relationships and split, it had nothing to do with me. At the time, however, he and Adam and much of their sophomore gang were all still naive enough to believe in the enduring power of hometown sweethearts. Sure, freshman year at Harvard had posed its challenges. But in general the friends you make freshman year tend to be friends of proximity: your assigned roommates, people who live in your dorm. You cling to them more out of necessity than actual compatibility. It's only later in college, with more security, more focus to your studies, larger dorm environments, and greater involvement in extracurriculars, that you actually find your real friends. And it's these people—some of whom are no doubt members of the opposite sex—who prove threatening to high school sweethearts. I was such a friend to Adam. Make no mistake, I wasn't threatening enough to kill his relationship completely—just to rough it up a bit. It later died on its own.

Adam and I started out as friends—me with a crush on one of his roommates, as I've mentioned, and him, conveniently enough, with a crush on one of mine. We worked on the same newspaper and hung out a lot before anything physical happened between us and even when it did it was hardly mistaken for the Fourth of July. We simply enjoyed the comfort of each other's company a great deal. When all was said and done we were friends who fooled around for about eight months, and it's possible that's a record. There are people who are friends who fool around for *years*, on and off, but we might take the highest honors for consecutive months. It's also possible, however, that we'd be disqualified since any number of people who knew us were under the impression that we were actually going out, which I can only take to mean that we were going about it all wrong.

When inquiring minds were informed that we *weren't* going out they wanted to know why not, and I can't say there weren't times when I didn't want to know myself. I mean I *knew* why. Her name was Sharon and she'd been going out with Adam for two or three years. She'd gone to France for a year and they'd agreed to see other people. What confused things was that Adam never seemed to see anybody but me. I, too, was allowed other interests but somehow Adam always took precedence. Looking back it was a pretty symbiotic relationship. In the absence of any worthwhile love interest in my life I still had the perks of having a boyfriend; we'd go to formals together, exchange backrubs, and basically bum around together all the time. And Adam had a close girl "friend" who could act like a girlfriend whenever he saw fit.

What should have been the best part about our arrangement for me was, of course, the fact that Adam had no interest whatsoever in having actual sex with me. Apparently *that* would have been a betrayal of his girl-friend. But what made things difficult was that Adam had a much better grasp on the "friends who fool around" concept—perhaps because his romantic life was already neatly packaged with Sharon's name on it, his picket-fence fantasies intact. Starved for romance, I wanted to know why Adam wouldn't give it to me. What was missing between us? What made her special? Wasn't he attracted enough to me to want to sleep with me? And since I func-tioned as a girlfriend, and was often mistaken for one, why was I being deprived of the title? I was doing all the work and all Sharon had to do was write the occasional letter and make the odd phone call.

The situation is not one I recommend and doesn't exactly do wonders for one's self-esteem. Just like busting your ass as the underling of someone who does no work and makes twice as much money as you do, playing second fiddle to a guy's actual girlfriend just feels wrong. It's an addictive situation, however, and when I was in it, it mattered less that I had no interest in having sex with Adam than it did that he wasn't interested in having it with me. Sure, I was glad to be free of the pressure, but not being wanted for sex was still a blow.

The fact that Adam had had sex with his girlfriend and didn't want to do it with me put me on a lesser plane. Instead of recognizing a bad situation and hightailing it in the opposite direction, however, I was challenged by the idea of making Adam wake up to what he was missing. Mind you, I wasn't going to give it to him if he ever came to want it. But even though I knew he wasn't the guy I'd settle down with, that we weren't "in love" by any stretch, the idea of someone's not wanting to have sex with me was hard to get a handle on, having encountered in the past couple of years a lot of men who did. The whole routine—man making advances, Tara setting limits—was becoming so natural to me that having a line drawn for me was jolting, regardless of whether the line was exactly where I would have drawn it myself.

Looking back I think the whole Adam thing gave me some insight into what drives men away from virgins—not insight into why someone like Cadman ran scared, but into how the word *no* can cause some difficulties in a relationship. When you're the person being rejected it's almost impossible to see that someone's decision to not have sex with you has less to do with you and your desirability than it does with that person's personal integrity or beliefs. If someone only wants to have sex with someone who is incredibly special to them and doesn't have sex with you, the natural assumption to make is that you're not special. Or not special enough. Unless you have more intuition and self-esteem than most people I've met in my time on this planet, you have no way of seeing that someone's decision to not sleep with you might really have nothing to do with you. (No offense.) It's hard to accept that someone can have a part of him- or herself—a part the individual is not ready to give up—that's more important than you are. Without question.

When put in the position of rejectee myself, I was torn. On the one side I was confident enough that I deserved better treatment, someone who loved me completely, to want to tell Adam to fuck off. I tried that a couple of times unsuccessfully; he was, after all, one of my best friends. The other side of me respected Adam's choice but needed reassurance not only that I was lovable but that I was sexually desirable—in spite of his rejection, in spite of my virginity. Because when you're a virgin, no matter how enlightened you are, you have vague memories of a playground bully who said he could tell whether girls were virgins by the way they walked, and carry with you a ridiculous fear of being found out. When you get dressed up a bit sexy to go to a party or club you're inwardly convinced you look like a poser. You may *feel* sexy, but you wonder whether you *look* like the grown equivalent of a little girl with her mother's lipstick smeared over her mouth, tripping in oversized high heels.

I won't blame the thirteen Barbie dolls I had growing up. Or the cosmetics ads and pretty faces in the magazines I read as a teen. But when you've had your share of lewd remarks from men on the streets and just as many dates with men who behave no better in the bedroom, it warps your views on such matters. If, apparently, anyone and everyone has the right to see you as a sexual object and say so, how do you see yourself as anything but? So when you encounter so many men who apparently would have no qualms about having sex with you, the ones who don't want to do it leave you a bit taken aback.

Sure, Doug and I had been together for nine months without any major protests on his part, but he'd also given me that line about my making a better wife than girlfriend, and we all know what that means. Likewise, Cadman had no problem fooling around with me now and then, but he'd no interest in having sex with me—at least not once he found out that it might actually *mean* something. Combined with the bizarre relationship I had with Adam, I was left asking myself what on earth men wanted and how I could possibly be it while at the same time remaining true to myself. There were men who would have had sex with me, but only on their own terms; men who couldn't handle my terms and therefore didn't want me; and now I'd been introduced to a man who didn't want me—at least not completely—because he was getting it else-where. What was a girl to do?

I knew I was attractive and had a lot of other things going for me, and I sometimes imagined that if I would only go all the way I would be any number of guys' dream girlfriend. But imagining myself as someone who had intercourse as a matter of course, saw it as a natural pro-gression in any relationship and granted it no "undue" significance, was about as hard as imagining myself with long, curly blonde hair and a D cup.

Somehow it just wasn't me.

And gosh darnit, I liked me. So the task at hand, I real-ized, was not merely finding someone who liked me; that hadn't proved too difficult. But finding someone who *was* like me. Convinced I wasn't going to find that person at Harvard—where I'd never felt like I'd found more than a handful of kindred spirits—I felt my graduation couldn't come soon enough. Rejected by fellowships committees and overlooked by Cabot House administrators for my extensive house committee work when class awards rolled around, I felt jilted all around by my soon-to-be alma mater. My pride at commencement didn't stem so much from having earned a Harvard degree as from my decision to enter a field—music journalism—in which a Harvard degree matters less than whether you remember who sang "Funkytown" or "Tarzan Boy" and when.

I can't say I was particularly proud of the fact that my virginity was graduating with me in spite of statistics to the contrary. I'm not sure I even thought about it. But I was damn sure I hadn't met the man of my dreams in college and glad of it. With my life truly my own for the first time ever, and completely left to my own devices, I was suddenly reminded of how much else there was to do.

Intercourse would have its day, but I was going to have mine first.

cHAPTER
10

I *don't know how I ever talked Carolyn into it.*
We were sitting in a bar at John F. Kennedy
International airport, with our fathers, waiting to board
Aer Lingus flight EI-106 to Dublin, via Shannon. The
length of our stay: anywhere from three months to a year,
depending on how things went.

My dad, no longer the intimidating figure of my child-
hood, was getting into the spirit of things as he and I
ordered our third "Big Beer" (twice as much beer as the
regular size for only a buck more). Carolyn's dad was
more concerned with whether or not he could get take-
out next door at Pizza Hut and bring it over to the bar,
not to mention where I had come up with this cocka-
mamie Ireland idea in the first place.

This was pretty indicative of the whole affair. My dad

had never questioned the validity of my jetting off to Dublin to try to start my career as a music journalist. He hadn't even once tried to tell me that going off to Europe was a lame excuse for not finding a real job or that I had simply seen *The Commitments* too many times. That it would pass.

To be honest, I *had* seen *The Commitments* too many times (three, to be exact) and had been fantasizing about this trip for almost two years. By my senior year in college, I'd become such a cheerleader for Irish rock that you'd have thought any number of Dublin bands had me on their payroll.

Carolyn's dad had made a point of mocking the very adventure I'd dreamed up by announcing at Carolyn's graduation party that his daughter, who had just graduated from Cornell, and her friend who had just graduated from Harvard, were going to Dublin to become waitresses. This was only partially true, because I'd made a contact at *Hot Press* magazine—Ireland's *Rolling Stone* equivalent—and my job prospects there looked good. But to Mr. Murray, I was Carolyn's weird and wacky friend, the kind of girl best avoided if you ever want to have a savings account.

In truth, we could have been more prepared. It was only when a bus left us in the center of Dublin, as we were looking through our bags for a map, that we realized a little research might have come in handy. Right about now. Knowing that there was a river dividing the city and that you didn't want to be looking like a lost tourist on one side of it would have been good. Knowing that that side was the north side and that we were on it would have been better.

Had we consulted a map earlier, we wouldn't have ended up dragging our suitcases (Carolyn's didn't even have wheels) down a number of very long blocks along the Liffey to a hostel, learning to our embarrassment along the way that the word *quay* refers to a strip of land along a river and is pronounced "key"—not "kway." If we had had any common sense whatsoever we would have had the foresight to invest in either backpacks or (knowing us) a taxi ride.

We finally arrived at our chosen hostel and asked the guy at the front desk for a private room. As he scanned the list of available rooms I realized that I had hooked up with him while visiting Noel on Long Island one summer's night a year earlier. In an overcrowded beach house, we'd shared a couch, some kisses, and maybe a little more. I asked him if he knew Noel Miller and had spent a summer in Montauk. He did and had, but didn't quite remember me so I didn't mention the couch.

Carolyn and I climbed three flights to our room and, with blatant disregard for the laws of jet lag, went to sleep.

We would stay somewhere else tomorrow.

Blast from my past aside, one night at the hostel convinced us of what we had already suspected—that we didn't like hostels and liked backpackers even less. We got into a cab, checked into Mrs. Bartlett's Bed & Breakfast, and spent the afternoon on the pay phone, calling ads in the paper regarding apartments. For a while it seemed we would never find a place, simply because we couldn't figure out the phone. It was one of these strange devices that still plague parts of Ireland; you have to wait until the person you're calling picks up before you insert your coin. Anyone who has used this kind of phone will know that all conversations conducted on one start off with at least a few seconds of unnecessary panic: *Will they pick up, won't they pick up, drop the coin NOW!* Carolyn and I sacrificed most of our change to Telecom Eireann before perfecting our technique.

When we finally got the hang of it and set about the task at hand, we found a room available just around the corner. We walked over and were given a tour by an incredibly good-looking Irish medical student named Aidan. To this day Carolyn refers to him as "Liquid Metal Man" since he looked like the villain in *Terminator 2*.

Carolyn and I would have to share a very small room, but the house itself was nicer than anything I had imagined we'd find. The green "tile" carpet in the kitchen didn't quite match the blue plaid wallpaper, nor did the brown flowery couches complement the pink wall-to-wall rug in the living room, but everything looked fairly new and clean. After spending a while in Ireland, the natives' profound lack of interior decorating skills would become more obvious to me; compared to a few others I encountered later on, this house deserved a color spread in *Good Housekeeping.*

Aidan himself lived there, and two other guys—one from France and one from Germany—would be moving in for the summer later that week. We told him we'd let him know if we wanted the room at around 6 o'clock the next evening when Aidan knew he'd be home to take our call. We looked at another room that afternoon, but the older woman in charge of the house wasn't half as sexy as Aidan. We said we'd let her know the next day, too.

That night, as we lounged on our lumpy B&B beds, watching with disgust the flies that were hovering around the hanging lamp in the middle of an otherwise pleasant room, Carolyn and I reviewed the situation. It was a pathetic conversation, really, both of us worried about what our families would think of us living with three guys, both convinced that the two we hadn't met would be rapists. Nails were bitten (actually, Carolyn polished hers), tears were shed, and sleep was hard to come by. This whole thing was beginning to feel like a mistake.

The next day, we were kicked out of our B&B when Mrs. Bartlett herself needed to head into town to do her shopping. A kind woman, she offered us a lift to our new home around the corner. We accepted, the only problem being that it was three o'clock—not six—so we hadn't told Aidan that we had decided to take the room. He was understandably confused as he opened the front door and eyed our luggage. Luckily he hadn't rented the room to anyone else, and we were able to move in right then and minimize our embarrassment. And fortunately we only had to live in fear of our imaginary housemates-from-hell for a few days. Ironically, Aidan ended up being the worst of the three guys in the house. Call him the devil we knew. I ended up going out with him . . . and he ended up dumping me big time.

Aidan and I first got together on an incredibly rainy night in Galway. Carolyn, myself, and my college roommate Catherine, who was visiting, had embarked upon a hitchhiking tour of Ireland. We'd coordinated our plans with Aidan, who had planned a gathering with his friends in Galway, and decided that we'd all meet at the King's Head for a few pints. Aidan and I were both in particularly sarcastic moods and were flirting like crazy throughout the evening. At closing time we all decided to go to a nightclub, and Aidan and I kissed for the first time while waiting for a taxi that'd take us there. The night was all downhill from there, and in many ways, so was our relationship.

When the club closed, there were no taxis to be found. Catherine and I started walking "home" and it promptly started pouring. We were soaked to the bone by the time we got to our B&B, which wasn't really a B&B at all. Since all the hostels in town were booked, an enterprising hostel owner had offered us three girls the converted garage of his home.

Carolyn had gone off with Aidan and his friend Ronan to sleep near the beach and watch the sunrise, but because of the rain and ensuing mud they couldn't pitch their tent. Genius that she is, Carolyn decided to bring them back to our room, convinced that if we all got up and cleared out early enough everything would be fine. When we awoke to the tea-bearing female head of the household knocking on our door at 8 A.M., it was pretty clear everything wasn't going to be fine. She saw male bodies on the floor and threw a complete shit fit.

"What, in God's name are these, these, these *men* doing here?" She acted as if she'd have to wash her mouth out with soap. "I demand an explanation."

I had a hangover not to be toyed with and since none of this was my fault, I waited to see how Carolyn would handle the situation. At last she spoke, in a blatant New York accent: "This is my brother and his friend. They couldn't put up their tent or find a place to stay. I didn't know what to do. I couldn't just leave them out in the rain."

The woman was not impressed, especially because when she demanded fifteen pounds from each of the guys for the pleasure of sleeping on her floor, they objected in thick accents. *Irish* accents. It was pretty clear that if Carolyn was, indeed, related to either of them, that their family was pretty fucked up and not worthy of staying in her house anyway. She shouted and shouted at Aidan and Ronan to get up and out, and when Ronan said that he was only wearing his underwear and that he didn't think she'd appreciate the view if he got out of his sleeping bag, she was visibly shaken.

"You just better get out of here because my husband's on his way home and he'll kill you. He really will. He'll kill you."

I didn't doubt it for a second—not if he was half as psychotic as she was. Still, I felt sorry for the woman, not to mention myself or the three English girls who were sharing the room and were just trying to get a decent night's sleep.

Then psycho-woman turned on Carolyn: "You've got *nerve* coming over here and bringing *strangers* into my house! We would *never* treat you with such disrespect, come to your country and *lie* like that!"

I didn't think it'd be wise to start quoting figures about illegal Irish immigrants in the United States. The way I saw it, it would have been best to pay the poor woman for her troubles and be on our way. Aidan and Ronan were being assholes. They gave the woman a few pounds, saying it was all they had, and I ended up forking over the rest. I wasn't about to let a little scene like this ruin my fledgling relationship, however, so I did my best to laugh along with the others as we walked back into town to hitch our next ride and part ways with Aidan and Ronan for the time being.

It was by no means a fairytale beginning, but Aidan and I ended up going out for a few months anyway. There was no great love between us, though I would have made you believe otherwise at the time. All that our relationship really consisted of was going out to a local pub, Slattery's, for a few drinks and fooling around when we had the time. I'd started working at the Rock Garden, a now-defunct restaurant-bar-club, and used to go home right after work every night just because he would be there—declining invitations to go for drinks with coworkers who would later become much more important in my life than Aidan had ever been. I wore makeup and perfume around the house all the time, fearful of revealing my natural self to a man whose good looks intimidated me.

For a while, at least, we plodded along as a couple—eyeing each other across the dinner table during nightly discussions of the English language (and which of us spoke it better) with Paul, our cute and almost lovable French housemate, and Cristoff, the German, and one of the most difficult people I've ever met.

In truth, much of the strain of talking to Cristoff came from the knowledge that he was constantly analyzing what you were saying and how you were saying it. Whether it was lessons in the pronunciation of a word as simple as *hot*, or pointless queries into the relationship of *mug* (as in coffee mug) to *muggy* (as in humid) to *mugger* (as in a thief), talking to Cristoff was a chore.

All that aside, Cristoff had technically rented a room in the house before Carolyn and me, so he was allowed to stay there when the house's real tenants returned from summer break. I, on the other hand, had to otherwise occupy myself until Cristoff went back to Germany and I could move back in. Carolyn, who missed her boyfriend and was running out of money, had decided to head home to New York.

A Canadian named Lorraine, who had come into the Rock Garden countless times looking for a job, offered me a couch in her place for the two weeks leading up to Cristoff's departure. She was a strange girl, waving all sorts of feminist flags while complaining with desperation about the lack of a man in her life. And since she presumed that any other woman her age would be as sexually indiscriminate and active as she was, I let her believe that I was fucking Aidan's brains out.

I'd had a lot of experience with this white lie thing. Another circumstantial friend whom I spent a lot of time with one summer once complained that she hadn't had sex in a really long time. I simply said, "I know what you mean." I thought it was easier for everyone; that way no one had to think of me as some pathetic, prudish freak and I didn't have to explain that I'm not.

So Aidan and I had decided that we'd use the time while I was out of the house to "date," to actually go out and do things instead of just fooling around. We planned to meet Friday after work for a few drinks at the downstairs bar at the Rock Garden. Pretty ambitious, eh?

I got off work at around twelve and got all dolled up waiting for Aidan, who was working part time at an "Italian" restaurant (the Irish put Cheddar cheese in lasagne) across the street. I went all out—new dress, nail polish, lipstick, you name it—and while pretty much every male employee at the Rock Garden noticed, Aidan didn't. He showed up in his food-stained work clothes to tell me that they had a lot of cleaning up to do and probably wouldn't be finished for around forty-five minutes, after which he'd be just as happy to go home if it was all the same to me.

Trying not to cry, I told him that I'd really been looking forward to seeing him. He said he just wasn't in the
mood. I went upstairs and muttered a few obscenities
including, "What a prick!" to fellow employees. Colin
started laughing and said "What'd you say? He's got a big
dick?" but I wasn't amused. I had a quick cry in the bathroom, consoled by Colin's girlfriend Sarah, before realizing I had an excuse to go talk to Aidan. I'd left my black
jeans, part of the Rock Garden "uniform," in the house
by accident and he had brought them into work for me.

I really needed them, and in truth I thought maybe
these five minutes had given Aidan time enough to realize what a big mistake he was making. I went across to
Paddy Garibaldi's, which was closed. Someone let me in
and told me Aidan was upstairs. He was upstairs, alright,
but not (as you or I might have thought) scrubbing tables,
mopping floors, or hunched over a calculator balancing
his checks or tips. No, he was yapping away with some
coworkers, glass of wine in hand and less than thrilled to
see me.

He gave me my jeans and I asked him if he were me if
he'd be very pissed off right now. He said he might be,
yes, and asked me to call him tomorrow. I said that I
might and might not, and returned to the Rock Garden
where I cried my eyes out as Sarah reminded me of all the
negative things I'd said about the relationship earlier that
week. When I was feeling better we got stoned. (Or was
that the other way around?)

Not only was I stupid enough to call Aidan the next

day, I was stupid enough to invite him to Lorraine's and offer to cook him dinner. He ate well. So much so that the leftovers I was hoping to save for Lorraine didn't exist. And when he said he'd do the dishes later, we retired to the living room. There, we sat on opposite sides of the couch, leaning only close enough to look at the pictures Carolyn had sent me of our hitchhiking journey. Aidan had been thoughtful enough to bring me the birthday package Carolyn had sent, if not thoughtful enough to buy me a present himself.

After the pictures, and annoyed at this opposite-side-of-the-couch thing, I started getting really obnoxious about the previous night's episode, pretty much begging for him to break up with me and get it over with. For some reason, I knew he had to be the one to do it. I had invested a lot of hope in him, you see. Stateside friends heard nothing but good things about him—good-looking, med school, funny—and at least one friend was sure I'd lose my virginity to him.

I'd thought about it, of course. We were *living* together, after all. So we weren't really sharing a room, let alone a bed, but it was pretty damned close. And wasn't that what people who lived together did together? Wasn't that the point? And wouldn't that just floor everyone at home—Tara moves halfway across the world and loses her virginity to a stunning Irish medical student she's living with and lives happily ever after. God, how I loved the idea of it. It sounded so . . . so, I don't know, *mature* or something.

And, on top of it, he was *almost* a virgin himself! He'd

had sex only with one girl before and said he regretted it since it was a drunk one-night stand with a girl he didn't particularly like. He sincerely seemed to wish that he'd waited for the right person to come along and acted, at least for a while, as if I were that person. But when it came down to his trying to have sex with me during a particularly hot session, I just couldn't go through with it. I have this terrible knack for knowing when men really aren't in love with me, and when I'm not really in love back. If it hasn't surfaced at some other point in the relationship, pressure from a carefully placed penis usually does the trick.

Back on my side of the couch, all I needed was a little bit more of the typically insensitive asshole male behavior I'd seen the night before to free me from Aidan's clutches forever. I didn't have to wait long . . .

Aidan just didn't enjoy being around me as much as he used to. He knew he'd regret breaking up with me later, but right now he felt like he wanted to be able to go out with the lads and not feel responsible to me for his actions. He would like it very much, of course, if we could still be friends.

I didn't really want to be his friend, and he knew as well as I did that friends in this case meant "not enemies," not "bosom buddies." Usually you only say that you don't want to be someone's friend in these kind of breakup situations because you still want to be something *more* than friends and think that if you stick to your guns, you'll get it. In reality you'll settle for friendship if refusing to means not having them in your life at all.

In Aidan's case, I'd become so convinced on a certain level that I just fundamentally didn't respect the guy that I really wanted nothing more to do with him. Suddenly, with perfect recall, conversations we'd had over the past months reeled through my head and all of the naive, simple-minded things he'd said to me rang out loud and clear. I'd overlooked far too much for far too long for the sake of a romantic adventure, and there would be no more denying it.

Aidan said he should probably go and I agreed. As he walked to the door, he actually said that I'd be able to move back into the house in a week or so and that I could call to find out the exact day of Cristoff's departure. When I said I'd probably find a new place to live he looked sincerely surprised.

"Are ya sure?" he asked, eyebrows raised as he unlocked his bike and rolled it toward the street.

I told him I'd think about it while I did the dishes.

cHAPTER

11

There are places you will live in your life that will attract houseguests in large numbers. Dublin, I quickly learned, is one of them. So is San Francisco, apparently. Omaha, from what I hear, is not. And neither is New Jersey—unless you have a lot of friends who have the misfortune of not knowing anyone who lives in New York.

Dan, a friend from college who would never be more than a friend, wrote me soon after I arrived in Ireland to tell me he wanted to visit. I had a hunch he was coming over with hopes that Ireland's dramatic cliffs and rolling hills had unleashed in me a deep-seated desire for him that Harvard's ivy walls had kept under wraps and figured it was only fair to give warning. So when I wrote back to tell him he was more than welcome, out of courtesy I slipped in the fact that I was going out with an Irishman. The day Dan mentioned as his probable arrival date passed without further communication and I felt my suspicions had been confirmed.

I got another letter a few months later, and right around the time Aidan dumped me, Dan and a woman who I think he wanted me to believe was a romantic interest of his—and maybe she was, who am I to say?—arrived in Ireland. I don't recall how we kept ourselves entertained for the duration of his stay, but when I introduced Dan to a bunch of friends from the Rock Garden he was less than impressed. Writing off the crowd I'd come to know and love as cliquey and self-absorbed, Dan didn't strike me as an especially pleasant guest.

He himself had spent the better part of a year living in Dublin and, from what he told me, it sounded like he had a lot less fun than I did. Upon this, his first return visit, he had few friends to see and it's possible he resented me for having gained both social acceptance and gainful employment with relative ease. The week before he arrived, I'd landed my own column at *Hot Press*, where I was working in addition to the Rock Garden; he'd spent his time abroad washing dishes.

We'd met as seniors at Harvard. Emma and I were booking bands for Friday night parties at Cabot House, and Dan called up looking for a gig. We talked a couple of times before we actually met, and both of our imaginations ran wild as any healthy and single imaginations would have under the circumstances. He *sounded* cute, whatever that's worth, and we seemed to have no shortage of things to talk about, so when we realized we were both planning on going to see Buffalo Tom, we decided to meet at the club. He'd be wearing a Harvard baseball hat, he told me—backwards.

The second I saw Dan across the semi-crowded floor at the Channel club, I took a good hard look around for other Harvard baseball caps. I knew that instant that we would never be romantically involved. "It"—that all-important spark—just wasn't there. It wasn't that he was ugly or anything. He's actually pretty cute. But as we all know, that's not always enough. Still, the fact that there was no great passion between us didn't stop me from hanging out with him, having lunch now and again, going to the odd gig, and inviting him to parties. It wasn't the kind of friendship that I thought would naturally spawn transatlantic visits, but Dan was far from the most random person to visit me, nor was he the rudest. Ann Marie, whom I'd worked with one summer, came to visit via Paris for a weekend and spent less than five minutes in my new flat before asking whether I'd be offended if she got a hotel room.

I was by no means living in the lap of luxury, but the starving-writer-living-abroad shtick had its appeal for me. The flat I'd found in the wake of my breakup with Aidan was in a borderline seedy part of town, and I was sleeping on a twin mattress that you could feel the floor through. It was upstairs from an "early house," a pub that opens at 7 A.M., which meant that I and my revolving door of flatmates could enjoy draught Guinness in the comfort of our own home at pretty much any hour. It also meant that at least once a week, when there was live music downstairs, I'd toss and turn for hours only to wake with "Sweet Caroline"—imagine an off-key Neil Diamond with a brogue—running through my head. My bedroom window was painted shut, my hairdryer doubled as a heater, and until one of my Irish friends sat me down and gave me a talking-to, I'd no idea that those people hanging out on the corner opposite ours were dealing drugs.

In truth, it was probably the bathroom that tipped the scales in favor of an en suite room in a B&B for Ann Marie. We shared the loo with our neighbor Jim. Chances are it was the toilet fur (picture the edge of a swamp) that sent Ann Marie off in search of tourist board–approved accommodations and I was just as glad. Four days later I put her in a cab for the airport and we haven't spoken since.

Dan had the good sense to check into a hostel before he even glimpsed the toilet. I think even he knew that we weren't *that* close—that staying with me might not be the most comfortable situation in the world. In truth, there was, by this point, almost palpable tension between us. Toward the end of senior year, Dan had invited me to a formal dance. I accepted—maybe I was trying to make up for the way I treated a harmless guy who asked me to his senior prom when I was a freshman—and spent a night being twirled and hurled around at the end of Dan's arm in our pathetic attempt to dance to a swing band, cringing with fear that my dress would rip at the armpits. At night's end he presented me with a dozen red roses and a wish that he'd met me earlier on in college. He expressed some pretty strong feelings for me that night—feelings I simply didn't reciprocate—and said that he wished there was more time for us to spend together.

I guess this visit to Dublin was his way of making time, though I'm not sure we spent it how Dan would have liked. Arguing about a talking Barbie doll wasn't exactly my idea of a good time, either.

The doll said "Math is hard" apparently, and some women's groups in the States were up in arms about it, Dan told me. Siding with the talking Bimbo, he argued that math *is* hard, and that there's nothing wrong with a doll saying so. My point that G.I. Joe would never admit to having trouble with algebra was lost on him.

Perhaps it was just that the Barbie thing put me on edge, but when talk turned to more serious topics— namely political correctness, AIDS, and sex—I found myself downright confrontational. Dan, as it turned out, was a virgin and imagined that our shared lack of intercourse truly bonded us somehow. I've felt that kind of camaraderie with fellow virgins before, but Dan was different. As he went on and on about how the world would be a better place if there were more people "like us," I was suddenly aware of why virgins so often get a bad rap. Not only was Dan unbearably self-righteous—as many of the more vocal virgins in the media tend to be—but he appeared to be carrying around an enormous chip on his shoulder.

There will be people who accuse me of self-righteousness, though it's obviously hard for me to see why. Strange that something called self-righteousness is so hard to recognize in one's self. Sure, when a friend of mine told me he'd slept with his girlfriend after just a few weeks I was maybe a bit too surprised or horrified. But I knew he'd only had sex with one woman before and thought he might take his time. When he told me she was the one who really wanted to get on with it, I was probably more jealous than anything.

See, I've always liked the idea of being completely swept off my feet—like these two people very obviously were—and doing it without a second thought, convinced that current bliss would never end. I've never begrudged anyone who has sex with someone they think they want to spend the rest of their life with—whether or not that's the way it actually turns out—but rather envied them for their ability to live in the moment. I mean I never set out to be a virgin at the age of 25. And I often wonder if perhaps the idea of waiting until you're married belongs to another time, like my parents', when more people got married right out of college. When things were somehow simpler. No matter how strong my convictions are, I can't help but wonder at times whether it's really worth the wait when the wait has proved to be so long. Especially when there are ever-decreasing numbers of people around me who seem to think that it is.

But over the years I've had to accept that it's not just going to happen that way for me, that I'm not going to be swept away—at least it's not likely I'll be having sex, well, tonight, for example. I've been told I think too much, that it prevents me from enjoying the moment. But since my tendency toward hyperanalysis has saved my ass many a time, I've never been able to see it as a character flaw.

Since I've no intention of changing, sometimes, yes, it's hard not to wish there were more people who saw it my way—not because I'm convinced it's the absolute right way but simply because it's hard to be part of such a silent minority. To make it worse, even when virgins aren't a minority, we behave like one, pretending we've had sex in an attempt to belong, telling fibs to avoid the issue entirely. I believe so strongly that sexual intercourse is an act in which you give yourself completely to another person—an act not to be taken lightly—that it's impossible for me to have a relationship with someone who doesn't feel the same. I guess I sometimes wish there were more men for me to choose from. If all the single men in the world filled an ocean, I'm lucky if the ones I feel I have the potential to have a meaningful relationship with can coat the bottom of an inflatable kiddie pool. Obviously, this is not exact measurement, but Joe (you know, the one who spent a season on *90210*) is by no means your average Joe.

When Donna broke up with Ray and Joe entered the picture, I smelled a virgin. When he said grace at

Thanksgiving dinner I knew for sure. And when Donna decided—before she knew that Joe was a virgin—that she was going to do it with him, not because she felt she was ready but because she didn't want to lose him, well, there wasn't even a question in my mind. Donna wasn't going to blow it. Not on anybody. Not on prime time.

The whole Donna-Joe thing is actually every virgin's dream. You fall head over heels for a guy only to find out he too has been waiting—that he held out in other relationships, like you, because he knew you were out there, waiting for him. So far as I can tell, this is not the way it works in the real world. Finding people who see sex as an act of spiritual giving, something that shouldn't be separated from love, and possibly something to reserve for one person alone, has proved hard enough. Finding someone who has lived his life accordingly in spite of all the pressure there is on guys to have sex has turned out to be equally difficult. And finding one of *those* who has a healthy attitude toward sexual activities in spite of it all seems near impossible. Then there's the issue of falling in love with said person, and there's no guarantee. In the past five years, I've met only two men who I know are virgins. One was gay. The other was Dan.

I know guy virgins have a rough life, and I don't mean to be cruel to Dan. I just think he harbored a really unhealthy resentment toward society for making his road so hard and that his attitude gives virgins a bad name. He seemed fundamentally pissed off that the whole world didn't see things his way, and basically thought that if you got AIDS through sleeping around that you deserved it. I'll admit I'm more likely to give money to breast cancer research than to AIDS research, but that's not because I don't care; it's because my fear of one is simply greater than my fear of the other. I'm not convinced this makes me a bad person, just a pragmatic one.

To a degree we all buy into the idea that women who wait are innocent and sweet or, these days, just plain smart. With men, there's always the question of whether he's ever had the opportunity, and I'll confess I imagined Dan's state as more imposed than chosen. Not because he wasn't attractive enough to get a girl or anything, but simply because he seemed so pissed off about it. For all of my frustrations in dealing with the fact that I've never felt it was the right time to go all the way, a part of me has always felt it's something that made me different— something concrete that set me apart and not necessarily in a negative way. Like a tattoo on an obscure body part; something that gave me a heightened sense of self-worth and uniqueness whether anyone knew about it or not.

Perhaps virginity and tattoos have more in common than I'd ever realized until this moment. At the very least getting rid of them both often proves difficult and sometimes painful. And just as a skull and crossbones, an "I Love Mom," or a simple rose can mean different things to different people, I suppose the way we view our virginity—and the loss of it—is so unique to each of us that Hallmark could put out a whole line of cards for the occasion, ranging from "Happy Hump Day" to "We're sorry for your loss."

I imagine Dan saw his virginity as a crucifix—an actual cross to bear—placed on his arm where the whole world could see and pass judgment so long as he was wearing short sleeves.

Mine I was beginning to see as an anchor, perhaps hidden away on an ankle or butt cheek. Something that grounded me when other aspects of my life were up in the air, out of control. Something that would one day give way and (bear with me for a second) let me set sail.

And yes—at times—something that seemed like a real drag.

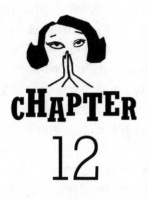

cHAPTER
12

Whoever said *"You can pick your friends, and* you can pick your nose, but you can't pick your friend's nose" didn't have very many friends.

At least not good ones.

It's never as simple as deciding, "I'm going to be friends with this person." Friends just happen—often completely randomly, often against our own will. Sometimes we feel blessed to have them; other times they're a pain in the ass and we wonder why we bother. But when it comes to our true friends, we have about as much say in choosing them as we do in picking out our own baby clothes.

And as for the nose-picking bit . . . I'm not sure any of my friends have ever picked my nose, but I wouldn't put it past a few of the ones I made in Dublin. I had the great fortune of falling in with an especially nice, especially fun crowd of people who worked at the Rock Garden, people whose lives I took great interest in while they in turn took an interest in mine. While my visitor Dan thought them cliquey, I never got that impression, but perhaps that's because the group as I came to know it was only forming when I became a member of it. As friends, a bunch of us just clicked; maybe that makes you cliquey to people you don't click with.

Lorraine, whose couch and working fireplace had gotten me through some rough times, tried her damnedest to become a part of the whole Rock Garden scene though she was continually denied employment at the very place that bound us together. She'd stop by almost every day, right as the day shift ended, and tag along to wherever anyone happened to be going. After I'd had a day off or skipped a night at the pub, I'd be caught up on the evening's events at work the next day. "Your friend Lorraine was there," someone would add as an afterthought.

You never really knew when or where she'd turn up, but one night, anxious to head out for a few drinks and lacking an accomplice, I was counting on her to stop by. We ended up heading over to the Norseman, just the two of us, where it became clear that our conversation was going to deteriorate into boring accounts of Lorraine's unsuccessful job search. Not a minute too soon, I had the good fortune of spotting a familiar face at the bar. I'd met Robert only once, but in the brief time we'd talked, mostly about my work for *Hot Press*, he proved to be rather charming. He'd also been under the impression that my being engaged in deep conversation (about a book I'd never read but somehow managed to claim changed my life) with the late great Bill Graham, an eccentric, hyper-intellectual journalist twenty years my elder, meant that I was sleeping with him. Once that issue had been cleared up, Robert and I hit it off pretty well.

He and a friend of his, Stephen, joined me and Lorraine at our table. Stephen, it turned out, was cousins with a guy in a band from Canada, and Lorraine had hooked up with one or two members so they started up a "small world" conversation. Robert and I found our own common ground. We'd both just been dumped. It was the start of a beautiful friendship, and maybe once or twice a little more than that.

In weeks to come, Robert, who deejayed at the Rock Garden and some other Dublin clubs, was always claiming to be a great cook and I told him I'd believe it when I tasted it. Unintimidated by what I claimed to be my discerning palate, he invited me to his place for dinner. We met up after work one evening and had a few pints before heading to Quinnsworth in Rathmines, where I'd shopped on a regular basis when I lived in that part of town. After collecting all the makings of a fine meal we headed for the beer section to top off our purchases, when who should be standing there selecting a case of Heineken but my former housemate Cristoff. He invited us back to the house for a few drinks since he was going home to Germany the following day, but I said I'd prefer not to tag along, 'cause, well, you know. Cristoff was insistent we come and assured me that Aidan himself was in the middle of moving out and probably wouldn't even be there. Robert eyed the beer and shrugged.

Back in the kitchen of my former home, beers in hand, all was going well until that all too familiar sound of a key in the front door—the sound that used to set my heart aflutter in expectation of the arrival of my loved one—revealed Aidan himself to be the key holder. Robert, bless him, answered questions like, "How do you two know each other?" with the perfect amount of affection and ambiguity, and when we left ("We should really go; I'm cooking Tara dinner and we've got all this food that should really be in the fridge.") I felt victorious. The look of (what I perceived to be) discomfort in Aidan's eyes, the fact that he couldn't bear to stay in the room and be social for more than three minutes, so fearful was he that I'd already found another, made me want to jump for joy. That is, until Robert and I actually did leave and instead of bursting into laughter I burst into tears. Robert did a good job of consoling me, not to mention feeding me. Such a good job that I ended up spending the night with him.

Robert already knew that I was a virgin so it wasn't an issue per se. He'd had virgins before, it turned out. A couple of them. And he wasn't particularly interested in having any more; at 30 he was getting a bit old for that. Likewise, my romantic interest in him was far from burning. When I'd first told Robert that I'd never had sex, he asked me if that's why Aidan had dumped me. Since the thought had never crossed my mind, the fact that it was the first to cross Robert's signaled to me early on that we weren't really on the same wavelength and would never make great bedfellows. At least not in the long run. Regardless, the morning after our fling, he'd tell me that when I did start having sex, I'd be damn good at it. An odd thing to say, maybe, but he meant it as a compliment so that's how I took it.

As for when I should actually start having sex, Robert always had something to say. If I expressed an interest in a new guy, he'd warn me to be careful. Then he'd turn around and tell me in the same breath that I should just get on with it. "It's like this," he began, during one of his more imaginative lines of argument. "Say there's this great mansion you live in with all these rooms and you hang out in each of these rooms at different times doing different things and they're pretty okay. But there's this one room with a lock on it. You have the key, but maybe you're nervous about what's on the other side. Then one day, just for the hell of it, you unlock the door and go in and see that it's pretty much like all the other rooms, just a little different, and maybe a lot cooler."

This reasoning, it must be noted, was coming from a man who told me he simply *can't* wear condoms (though he had no problem sleeping with three women in one week), and whose then-partner was close to a month late at the time. Still, he wasn't without his supporters as numerous other friends of mine, notably Colin and Sarah, suggested that maybe my time, if not my prince, had come.

Colin, who was undoubtedly the center of the Rock Garden group, is hipper than hip; an MTV veejay waiting to happen. He spends more time primping than his longtime girlfriend Sarah does and doesn't think there's anything strange about wearing leather pants and shades while hiking along a cliff on the west coast of Ireland on an overcast day. A barman by trade, he gets offered jobs in Dublin's trendiest pubs and clubs without asking and, unlike most men I know, is truly off when he's having a bad hair day. Better still, he actually *has* bad hair days. He's impossible to embarrass, mischievous in his pranks, and some would say vulgar in manner when discussing some of our less glamorous bodily functions.

Together he and Sarah, perhaps an odd match for Colin with her master's in economics and more sophisticated way, decided that I was brainwashed by my parents and the Catholic Church into believing sex is something special. By all indications, I'm an intelligent, independent thinker, so why won't I wake up to the fact that sex is really no big deal?

If I were Colin or Sarah, I probably wouldn't think sex was that big a deal, either. They basically grew up together, a few houses apart on the same street, and have been going out—on and off—for what must be close to seven or eight years now. They were each other's first and are now engaged to be married. If I'd fallen in love at age 16, had sex, and were still with that person today, I'd be as happy as a Saturn owner and probably wouldn't understand why someone might still be holding out at age 25 either. Not when my own experience with sex had been so good. Nonetheless, they'd argue and argue with me as though there were a $50,000 reward for information leading to the loss of my virginity, and settled for theorizing on my deeper motives once they were sure I wasn't so easily swayed.

There were other friends on my side, but they were mostly fellow virgins (Scott, a gay virgin, and possibly one of my favorite people on the planet, actually hugged me when I told him), so I was as surprised as anyone to have support for my choice to abstain come from a most unusual place, indeed a most unusual woman, Melanie.

Melanie (that's her real name, she insisted) just did things differently. An English black woman with short, kinky bleached blonde hair, she was already a bit of a novelty in overwhelmingly white Dublin when she came to work at the Rock Garden, and her style made her even more of one. If you thought long and hard, you'd have a hard time thinking of an instance in which you were sure she was wearing a bra, and if you had a particularly interesting or important conversation with her, she might bring you flowers the next day to say thanks. There was nothing she wouldn't say to your face (she told me she didn't like me at first simply because I was American), and somehow more she could find to say behind your back, but she wasn't what you'd call malicious. She had offbeat clothes to match her offbeat way and eyes so expressive that you would have thought her capable of making them jump out of their sockets if she was shocked.

But of course, nothing surprised Melanie, perhaps because there was almost nothing she didn't claim to already know. You could tell her your deepest, darkest secret only to have her respond, "I might have guessed as much" and tell you why rather convincingly. People who subjected themselves to her psychoanalysis would later relate what she'd said with a "Do you believe the nerve of her" tone, but the next day they'd be back for more.

So my virginity came as no surprise to Mel. Not that she'd pegged me for a virgin before she knew for sure, but once she found out (I don't even think I was the one who told her) she said it just made sense. I was a bit ticked that she claimed to be able to read me so well, and maybe on some level I'd kind of prided myself on being told by a fellow virgin, "You don't act like one," and was less than thrilled with the possibility that I hadn't fooled everyone I thought I'd fooled over the years. Things I'd said and done, things not even relating specifically to sex or virginity, had apparently given me away.

If Mel could see through me, maybe everyone could, I thought, and imagined myself the subject of great speculation in a neighborhood full of nosy housewives. The leader of the local gossip pack would eventually figure me out and invite her crew over for coffee and crumb cake to share the news.

"The McCarthy girl," she'd say leadingly. "Virgin."

Others present would nod their heads and exclaim, "That explains it!" as if they'd been trying to pinpoint the root of my peculiar habits ever since I moved in. "No *wonder* she doesn't have any kids," the simpleton of the group might offer, and I'd spend the rest of my life as the subject of knowing glances in the supermarket.

Melanie threw no such glances. As much as she claimed to have everyone figured out, she knew there was always more to know about someone, and we talked about sex and virginity frequently. To my own surprise, having thought I had Mel figured out to some degree myself, she told me she sometimes felt like a virgin herself in spite of the fact that she'd been with a number of men. On a spiritual and emotional level, she didn't feel she'd ever given herself completely to someone and, inspired by our talks on the subject, decided that waiting until she was truly in love again before having sex again might not be such a bad idea. A lot of people scoff at "born again" virgins or the idea of reclaiming your virginity, but if people decide that the way they've experienced sex before was not positive for them, more power to them if they have the will and willpower to change it.

Whether she was born again or not, finding an ally in Melanie, who fell head over heels for and married one of the next guys she dated, finally made me realize that lying about my virginity was pretty useless at this stage of the game. No one particularly cared one way or the other, and, in fact, people who I assumed would think me crazy might actually not feel so different themselves. Once, before I knew Colin very well and when I was still going out with Aidan, he asked me whether I'd had mind-blowing sex on Aidan's birthday. I lied, quipping "more than once," because there were four or five other people in the room who I didn't think really needed to know the real deal. Colin would give me enough shit for lying in months to come that I'd begin to see how fibbing could be more trouble than it's worth. The fact that he, Sarah, and Mel took me seriously—and that I'd been challenged by friends with a range of views on the subject and come out of it with my ideas intact—gave me courage enough to tell the truth, the whole truth, and nothing but.

Well, sort of. There were still times when bending the truth seemed like the easiest thing to do. I somehow got on the subject of sex with a musician I'd met in Belfast— okay, it was because we were in bed—and told him, in the course of our conversation, that I had had very few relationships involving sex in the past. (The mistress of understatement strikes again.) When he asked me playfully to tell him the strangest place I had ever had sex I was tempted to make something up but blanked.

"I can't answer that question," I began, "because I've never had sex . . ."

I thought as long and hard as you can in a split second about adding "in any strange places," which would have been a perfectly true statement. But I couldn't do it, so there it was, just hanging out there: "I've never had sex . . ."

Period.

"But you were just talking about relationships where sex had been involved."

Caught.

Ah, yes, I attempted, but only in the sense that it had been brought up, discussed, and decided against.

Bill concluded that my virginity was "interesting" because . . .

"Well, because you don't find too many virgins these days."

Right about now, I'm sure Bill, who'd told me earlier that he hadn't been interested in anybody in a really long time before meeting me, was probably pret—ty ticked off that of all the women in Belfast that night he had to pick a bleedin' virgin for what I'm sure was intended to be a one-night stand.

"What are you, saving yourself for marriage or something?" he asked, and all of a sudden—and maybe you're surprised it took me so long—I felt ridiculous.

Not because *waiting* was ridiculous, but because attempting to dodge the subject—a subject about which I obviously felt very strongly—was a ridiculous thing for me to be doing. And because lying in bed barely dressed beside a guy I barely knew was a ridiculous place for me to be. I *was* waiting for Mr. Right, and the odds of this guy being him were about a zillion to one. So as I told this stranger the whole truth and nothing but, that marriage wasn't so important to me as finding love, with a capital *L*, blah blah blah, it suddenly struck me that I was going about it all wrong. And had been for quite a while.

In truth, I was probably as close to a slut as a virgin can get. I had really high standards when it came to whom I wanted to spend my life with—and would talk about such matters among friends with great idealism and conviction—but I had incredibly low standards regarding whom I'd spend a night with. And I guess until now I hadn't realized that each night I spent with the wrong guy was one less I'd have with the right one. I knew I wouldn't necessarily find the right one tomorrow, but since I didn't feel particularly good about it when Bill completely blew me off a week later, I took my Cupid's arrow and decided to do something different with it for a change.

Aim high.

cHAPTER
13

At some point in our lives we all set our sights
on someone whom we believe to be, on some level, out of
reach. Maybe they're too cool, too good-looking, too
witty, too popular . . . too whatever you're lacking yourself. We truly believe, underneath it all, that if we could
break through those superficial things this person could
love us wholeheartedly forever. Or at least like us a little
bit. For a little while. That would be okay, too.

As a virgin, the whole "he'd never go for me" idea has
always had an added dimension for me—particularly
when faced with a male specimen who I'm convinced
would laugh in my face if he knew I'd never had sex. Men
who, because of their track record, know they can get it
whenever they like and therefore have no intention of
going without. Men who, by virtue of their being signif-

icantly older than I am, would be incapable of seeing me as anything more than moral jailbait if they knew my status. Unlike guys who don't want the responsibility, these men—and they're *men*, not guys—just couldn't be bothered. Not when there's hassle-free, guilt-free sex to be had elsewhere.

That's how I saw Simon, a manager—my boss!—at the Rock Garden. From the beginning I think there were levels on which we understood each other completely. I lied through my teeth to get the job, concocting an elaborate story about my experience waitressing at New York's Cafe Vivaldi, and Simon, sensing both the deception and the desperation with which I wanted to work at this hip and happening joint, hired me—not as a waitress but as a hostess. The job required little to no restaurant experience so long as you could think on your feet *and* stand on them for eight hours a day.

Since I'd never set foot in Cafe Vivaldi except to eat a piece of chocolate mousse cake, the job was as perfect for me as Simon's was for him. He was so completely cool in every way that it would have seemed an injustice if he'd ended up a bookkeeper or insurance salesman. He was English with a superb accent, funny, smart, caring, friendly, and incredibly witty. He had cool clothes, good looks, and an incredible body, and was truly great at his job. Pity, then, that when the Rock Garden met with some financial difficulties he was the first to be let go. The female staff members in particular mourned the loss of their most accessible manager, but none could deny that there was a flip side. Since Simon was no longer our boss he was available to us in a way he'd never been before. So began the battle for his affections, a battle in which I thought, in a twisted way, Simon himself was the enemy.

There were other enemies, too. Four of them to be exact. Melanie, Vanessa, Katrina, Caroline, and myself were all vying for Simon's attention one way or another (for that matter, so was Scott), and were all convinced that we were the one he really wanted, regardless of how things turned out. Melanie was just in it for sport, I think. She liked to analyze people, to figure out what made them tick; figuring men out often seemed to involve figuring out how to get them to want her, and no one could deny she had a knack for it. An informal poll of male staff members revealed Mel to be on the top of their most desirable fuck list. Vanessa, a virgin like myself, didn't put up much of a fight for reasons I understood; she and I were simply out of our league up against the likes of Katrina and Caroline. These were women who would stop at nothing for the sake of a man like Simon. They were good friends, but they weren't afraid to take the gloves off for a prize this great. As it turned out they would each have their chance with him, but not before I'd had mine.

In the Rock Garden gossip pool, there was much curiosity and speculation over what actually happened between Simon and me, so here it is for the record: not much. My line at the time, "We spent the night together," was both true and about as far from the truth as possible.

Not long after he'd left the Rock Garden, Simon made an appearance in the Norseman, where a number of us had gathered for a going-away party for a staff bartender who was moving to America. Simon and I were both in especially sarcastic and flirtatious moods—for me the two often go hand in hand—and weren't particularly interested in calling it a night at pub closing time. As much of the group dispersed, the decision was made to go bowling. To my surprise and pleasure, the late-night contingent included only Simon, myself, and the couple he'd been staying with ever since the bump in his career path forced him to relinquish his trendy flat. I'd been commissioned to deliver food from the Rock Garden to that flat one time when Simon was sick with the flu and had hoped a time would come when I'd be invited in for other reasons.

Situation as it was, I had to settle for an invite back to Eileen and Gerry's place where the four of us would get high and watch *The Good, the Bad, and the Ugly.* Or at least that was the plan; I'm not sure I really did either of those things. There was a joint being passed around, but I was paranoid about a cold sore I'd developed and wary of spreading germs. And I know I must have been focusing my eyes on the television as the film played, but I'd have a hard time writing a summary that would pass for a second grade book report. I was simply too preoccupied by the fact that I was sitting beside Simon.

Me and Simon.

Not Melanie and Simon. Not even Caroline or Katrina and Simon.

At least not yet.

No, none of them were there, and if they had been, they certainly would have been doing more than sitting. Feeling a bit silly as a virgin contemplating seduction, I just couldn't muster up the courage to make the first move, and apparently neither could Simon. When the movie was over and Eileen and Gerry were upstairs in bed, we switched to MTV and made it as far as reclining together on the couch. By the time we got to a little hand caressing, the release was so great and the hour so late I thought we'd collapse.

Outside of some kissing, a little involvement on the part of my breasts, and an abridged night's sleep on the living room floor, that was pretty much it. Simon declined an invite back to my place a few nights later, I went home to New York for the holidays, and I returned in two weeks to find that the man I'd spent my holidays longing for was sleeping with Katrina.

Vixens 1, Virgins 0

I suppose the best thing you can ask for in the face of such a defeat is the ability to convince yourself that you didn't really want to win anyhow. That came easily for me. Sure, I wanted Simon and liked the idea of being with him tremendously. But I knew he was the kind of guy who would wear down my defenses quickly; any scenario I imagined in which I was involved with him included things like living together and having sex—steps I simply didn't feel ready for yet somehow felt being with Simon would require. It was as if he already occupied the adult world I didn't feel I'd fully become a part of yet, and I was as drawn to that world as I was scared shitless of it. Sure, I was living thousands of miles away from home and making my own living, but in many ways I still felt like a kid. Simon could have taken advantage of that quite easily. At the time, the fact that he didn't almost made me want him more. If I'd been a different person he'd have been the man of my dreams.

Sometimes I really wanted to be that other person. There was something so *normal* about her. She talked about sex with her friends with ease, she didn't feel like a freak talking to her gynecologist, she had a diaphragm and some spermicide in her night table drawer, and could walk into a sex shop without feeling like a drug enforcement agent at a Dead show. She was everything I already was only better. Or at least better equipped to function on this planet with a minimum of hassle.

She probably would have won the battle for Simon. None of her friends would have had to try to convince her to sleep with him, as Colin and Sarah did with me, because she would have already done it and loved every minute. She'd have lost her virginity years ago under the best of circumstances with a long-term college boyfriend whom she eventually did the breaking up with and gone on to become a perfectly well-adjusted, sexually active woman.

But I am what I am, and was never very keen on the idea

of "losing" my virginity; the phrase implied a carelessness with which I simply couldn't see myself ever treating something like sexual intercourse. I could see "giving away" one's virginity, and had moments when I could see why people might want to "get rid of" it, but "losing" it I just couldn't fathom. Look up *lose* in a thesaurus and you find things like "suffer loss of," "be deprived of," "misplace," "miss," "confuse," "be the loser," "suffer defeat," "have the worst of it," and, my personal favorites given the context, "mislay" and "take a licking."

I wouldn't have minded taking a licking from Simon, but I was uncomfortable with the power his being seven years my elder granted him. I wasn't prepared to expose myself to someone who might laugh at me or condescend to me—to "lose" anything he might win—nor was I ready to undergo the metamorphosis needed to make me into the person I believed he would have wanted. I envied her at times, sure. But willing myself to become her was another thing entirely. For all I knew she had an abortion in her past or had contracted HIV. For all I knew, her sex life sucked. For all I knew, Simon would have rejected her, too.

He moved back to London in months to come and pursued a long-distance relationship—one that lasted longer than anyone would have suspected—with Katrina, who eventually moved to the States. Not long after Katrina had gone abroad, I had the chance to visit London with my college roommate Emma, who was studying at Cambridge for a year. We ended up crashing one night in Simon's flat, where we drank Champagne into the wee hours, shooting the breeze. Removed from the Dublin scene in which I'd seen him as a star player, Simon no longer seemed larger than life. Yes, he was the kind of guy who had Champagne in his fridge for no reason. Yes, he had a body to die for. But he was hardly the ruthless womanizer I'd imagined; my own innocent night with him should have told me that already. He spoke about Katrina with true affection, and it dawned on me that it wasn't the sex thing that kept him and me apart. Sex was most definitely a weapon, one I simply didn't have in my arsenal; I was as unprepared to rush into it for the sake of a guy I barely knew as I was to hold a loaded gun to my head. But the fact that other women had sex on their side didn't mean they'd always win. Or that that was *why* they won. Or even that I thought all of their battles worth fighting.

The sex issue had definitely kept me at a distance, but it hadn't kept me my from destiny. And as I bid Simon farewell, I didn't see him, as my wounded pride would have liked me to, as a fool who passed me up for the sake of a good lay, for a lesser woman. I saw a man whom I was fond of who I believe was fond of me, but more fond of someone else. And fonder still, eventually, of her best friend.

Things might have happened differently, and I might have become that other me. After all, *I* was the only thing keeping me from becoming her. Until now, I guess I hadn't realized how great a force I was to be reckoned with. The one thing I *did* know, and it's something that the man I met in the wake of my defeat at the Battle of Simon would teach me more than once, was that everything happens for a reason.

Or in my case, didn't happen.

cHAPTER 14

Every once in a while I still have dreams about him. Taken alone, that fact doesn't say a whole lot since I dream about anyone and everyone—even the oral surgeon who pulled my impacted wisdom teeth—at one time or another. But dreams about Nick are especially vivid, and it always takes me a while to shake the creepy feeling that I've just spent time in the company of someone I haven't seen in three years and may never see again. Someone who, insofar as it concerns me, might as well be dead. And not just because there were a couple of times when I might have wished him so.

In many ways, this was my fairytale relationship, my wildest dream come true. (Well, maybe not my *wildest*, but that involves me and *The X Files'* David Duchovny and a couple of limber aliens and I'd rather not get into it now.)

He was a really good-looking guy (at least I thought so), with the dark hair, crystal blue eyes, and tall, lanky build I'd always claimed were my type. He was Irish with the accent to prove it and shared almost all of my interests wholeheartedly. I'd spent years believing that somewhere out there, there had to be the male equivalent of me, and Nick seemed to be it. Equally at home at clubs and museums, he was the only guy I'd ever met who seemed truly to have been cut from the same mold.

I was so smitten that I fantasized about completely blowing America off in favor of a kinder, gentler existence in Ireland forever. This was a man for whom, at least for a while, I could see myself forsaking friends, family, and New York delis.

"*Him?*" you might say if you met him.

"*Really?*" you'd press, after spotting the butter on your wafer-thin Irish ham and cheese sandwich.

In truth, from the beginning there were things about him that drove me crazy, like the fact that he was way too mad about me way too fast, but I'd gotten used to that. When I fall for real I fall pretty slowly. I'd figured that out. So I stuck with it despite my wariness of men who are certifiably crazy about me from the start. I'd encountered too many who claimed to love me without even knowing me. And while all of them hadn't necessarily learned their lesson (that to know me is *not* necessarily to love me), I had learned mine: breaking up with these sorts is hard to do.

As I had hoped, after a few weeks with Nick those lit-

tle annoying things—his bad tooth, his jittery manner-
isms, his coffee and cigarette breath—actually became
endearing. Or at least I eventually decided to stop complaining about them, having accepted Nick on his own
terms and grown rather quickly to love and care about
him deeply.

We'd met because he managed a band whose demo
tape I'd given a great review. I listened to a lot of really
crappy tapes in my line of work—demos that demon-
strated nothing more than a complete lack of musical
skill or artistry—so when a thoroughly good one like
Crimplene's made its way into my Walkman it was reason
to rejoice. He called me up to thank me for the review
and asked me to come see the band live. We chatted after
the show and he offered me a lift home, but I declined. I
felt safe in Dublin, with its low crime rate, and often
found myself walking alone at night simply because I felt
I could; it's a luxury American women simply don't have.
Nick called me at work the next day to thank me again
for my interest in the band and to make sure I'd gotten
home okay. I had.

So began a telephone relationship of sorts. He'd call
me at work to ask for a plug for the band in *Hot Press*, and
each time we'd talk a little longer about something a little
less work related. An invite to lunch wasn't so long in
coming and a dinner invite followed quickly on its heels.
Somewhere in between asking me out and taking his seat
across from me at a table for two at Tante Zoe's, he found
the time to break up with his girlfriend of five years, who

I had no idea existed. Apparently, she was about as thrilled to find out about me as I was about her.

I suppose I should have been warned. I mean what kind of guy tries on a new love interest for size before resolving matters with someone he's been with for five years? But by the time I'd gotten the scoop on the ex, Nick and I already had two pretty stellar dates under our belt (not to mention a little action below the belt) and I was simply having too much fun.

On our first date, it was lashing rain and we were caught out after dinner without an umbrella. Huddled together under Nick's coat we made a dash for the pub across the road, where we sipped Guinness and talked about books, authors, and music, sharing bits of our life stories along the way. At pub closing, he dropped me home without so much as a kiss and I went to bed terribly impressed.

After date number two, all systems were go. We'd met before a gig for drinks, over which we pretty much established we could get married without either of us being disowned in the process. Not that we were hearing wedding bells just yet, but it was nice to know we agreed on all the big things (kids, husband-wife roles, classic rock . . .) before proceeding. After the concert, walking back toward town, he took my hand and sent tingles through every inch of me. I still remember how different the feel of it was—this new and mysterious hand in mine. How it felt in an instant as if I'd grabbed onto something I wasn't going to let go of too easily. And obviously I don't mean that literally. The kiss that followed a few blocks later was no less exquisite, and it was quickly decided that the taxi was making only one stop. My place.

It was most definitely love. What else could compel a difficult sleeper like myself to start sharing my mattress—my *twin* mattress, remember?—with anyone on a regular basis. I mean who can get any decent sleep that way? I've never been a touchy sleeper; spooning and cuddling is all well and good, but when it's time to actually sleep, a line down the center of the bed would serve me well. Preferably one that gives an electric shock to the man who dares put a knee or toe across it. If someone had asked me, "Did you sleep with Nick?" in those exact words, I probably would have said, unthinkingly, "Not particularly well." As Seinfeld has pointed out, sleeping with someone and having sex with them really couldn't have less in common.

He was in love, too. So in love that he couldn't believe he'd ever thought he'd been in love before. At least that's what the card he gave me for Valentine's Day some months later said. He liked watching me blow-dry my hair, which I had a lot more of at the time. He called my butt (which I also had a lot more of at the time, come to think of it) devourable and even thought my ankles were sexy. As we cruised through the Irish countryside on our romantic weekend getaways, it was all he could do to keep his hands—well, hand—off them. He was driving, and I'd be in the passenger's seat with my stocking feet perched on the glove compartment. He'd reach over to gently caress an ankle, I'd look over at him, and we'd smile. Corny couple moments were in no short supply. Maybe that's why no one could believe I still hadn't done the deed.

Nick had gotten a Morrison visa and was emigrating to Philadelphia after we'd been together for just a few months; since I'd made plans to move home to New York shortly thereafter, we'd no intention of letting the ocean between us come between us. Still, his move to the States was a big deal and at his going-away party at one of our favorite pubs Colin pulled me aside:

"Are you going to do it tonight?" he asked, tugging on my shirtsleeve excitedly. "I think you should do it."

Paula, a coworker some years older than me, was perplexed since it was apparently obvious to everyone that I was in love.

"Not even *Nick*?" she practically choked when I told her I'd never had sex.

"Do you have oral sex?" she asked a minute later and I nodded.

"You must be good at it," she assessed, exhaling a breathful of smoke out the side of her mouth. Then, after a contemplative moment: "He must be *dying* for it," and a pause. "He must be dying."

Well, if he was, there were certainly no visible symptoms. When I moved home to New York, Nick and I saw each other almost every weekend. We picked up right where we left off and left off where we used to leave off with no complaints on either side. We played strip poker, watched pay-per-view porn, even took a four-day trip to the Bahamas, and lack of intercourse notwithstanding Nick seemed to be the picture of health. He claimed, in fact, that his "sex" life had never been better. And when, after we'd been together for about a year, I asked him if he'd have sex with me if I wanted to, he said no. In every other relationship that he'd had sex in, they'd waited about a year and half, and Nick was determined to wait that long with me, maybe even until we were married.

Do you believe the cheek of him?

There I was, at the ripe old age of 23 thinking that maybe, just maybe, it was time to go for the gold, and the lucky guy I'd set my sights on had the gall to turn me down!

I understood the nobility of his intentions. I mean, all my life I'd been looking for someone who wouldn't pressure me. Someone whom I loved who loved me for me, regardless of whether I'd sleep with him. And here he was, in the flesh, saying that he himself wished he'd waited until he was married, regretted that I wouldn't be his first. So I'm not quite sure why once he said it—"I want to wait"—it wasn't exactly what I wanted to hear.

I guess a part of me didn't think he had any right to make that decision. Since he'd already had sex with other people before, I didn't think he had the right to *not* have sex with me if he claimed to love me more. It would take me a while to shake the idea that our having sex together should be my decision. That he was lucky I deemed him worthy.

I'm not sure I would have done it even if he *had* been game. Maybe I was just testing the waters. There were doubts in my mind that he was "the one" as much as I loved him. And I guess the fact that he didn't want to have sex with me made me wonder whether he was really sure about our future together. There were tinges of the old "if things don't work out . . ./I don't want the responsibility" shtick in his arguments for waiting, and that routine was wearing me down. I'd started to imagine that I'd know I'd found the man of my dreams when I came across a guy who didn't fear the responsibility (read burden) but one who embraced it. Someone who felt that it was his job to do it and do it right.

With Nick determined to prove he could wait and me feeling a bit dejected, the time wasn't yet right. And I guess the main reason we never had sex is that the right time never came.

Things started to deteriorate right around the time I'd finally gotten my act together and gone to a doctor who decided to remove a swollen gland in my neck. It had been there for over a year and I imagined that once I was cut open some horrific mutant alien was going to reveal itself—its tentacles firmly gripping my brain—and ruin my chance of ever having a normal life again. Hypochondriacal fatalist that I was in the lead-up to surgery, I was probably not the funnest of girlfriends for a spell. Still, for a man who claimed to love me so, Nick put on a particularly poor display. No flowers, no card, not even a fulfilled promise of a phone call the day after the procedure. He was a shit, basically, and it started to become a pattern.

Suddenly Philly seemed to be off-limits and Nick was so keen on coming up to New York on weekends I knew he was hiding something. He denied to the high heavens that there was someone else, but I still wonder whether there was someone he *wanted* to be someone else. Maybe he'd met her for lunch, but hadn't thrown out the dinner invite just yet, if you catch my drift.

In any case, lying in bed one September Sunday morning at my place, I asked Nick to tell me what was on his mind; he'd told me on the phone the previous week he had some things he wanted to talk about. On this morning, he said I should forget about it, that it wasn't important, but I pressed him. He'd assured me days earlier that it wasn't anything bad, so I inferred it was something good and couldn't have been more wrong.

While Nick used to think that he wanted to marry me, he no longer felt that was where our relationship was heading.

Just wanted me to know.

He wasn't exactly breaking up with me—at least he didn't think he was. He just wanted to give official notice that he was no longer 100 percent sure he wanted to settle down with me. Mind you he would be perfectly content to continue going out with me.

Upon interrogation, Nick just didn't think he wanted the pressure of our relationship anymore and needed time to think about it. Ultimately, he broke down, crying in my arms telling me how much he loved me. He was sorry he hadn't really said or shown it lately. I cried my eyes out (and again, I don't mean that literally) as I watched him walk to his car from my corner window.

I've Liz Phair to thank for preparing me for what I imagined would be a long and difficult talk with Nick about the future of our relationship—or lack thereof. Deciding that, while Nick was "thinking," a change of scenery was in order, I phoned up my college roommates, who were all still living in Cambridge. Having secured three sympathetic pairs of ears for the weekend, I borrowed Dad's second car and hit the road. I spent the four-hour drive to Boston (*and* the one back) listening to Phair's *Exile in Guyville* over and over and over again. With all of its life-affirming, self-affirming, make-him-jump-through-hoops-for-you talk, it's perhaps the best being-dumped soundtrack ever recorded. So after about twelve times through I was prepared for anything.

A wonderful night out with an incredibly attractive man the same weekend probably worked just as many wonders. It was a completely platonic night—at least nothing nonplatonic actually *happened*. He was, after all, another of those significantly older, unabashedly virile men whose sexual power set my virgin knees knocking, and besides he had a girlfriend. We had dinner, went to a bar looking out on the Boston skyline for drinks, walked along the Charles River, and strolled around the fountain near the Christian Science Monitor complex. Talking about love and life until three in the morning with a man who was both incredibly insightful and forthcoming with his feelings put the whole Nick thing in perspective. There I was, baring my soul to someone who until then had basically been an acquaintance, and he was baring his back in a way Nick just wasn't capable of. There had been life before Nick, I was reminded, and there would be life after him. Maybe that was even what I wanted.

Despite my efforts in coming weeks I never saw Nick again. He agreed to come resolve things face-to-face one Saturday and never showed. When I asked him why he bagged he made up some lame excuse. When I asked him why he hadn't called to *tell* me his lame excuse, it was all I could do not to laugh.

"I meant to," he practically whimpered.

I was no fool. And I knew Nick well enough to know how he could be. "Nick's coming here on Saturday to talk things out," I'd written in my journal, "*or so he says.*" Though I'd hoped for more from a man I'd shared my life with for over a year, a man to whom I believed I'd been a good friend, I'd prepared myself for the worst and gotten it.

"I hope everything works out for you over here, Nick," I said, because in spite of everything I really did. And then, my practiced line delivered, I hung up.

As much as I'd prepared myself, I couldn't believe it had come to this and was more hurt than I'd ever been in my life. The only way I could see to come to terms with the situation in the days and weeks that followed was to convince myself that Nick himself was so upset that things weren't going to work between us that he couldn't bring himself to look me in the eyes and tell me it was over. I had to convince myself that he was simply weak— not malicious—and that I wouldn't have wanted to spend forever with someone so cowardly.

The last time I'd been intimate with Nick had been particularly, well, intimate. This doesn't surprise me—I think we sometimes try to compensate for what's lacking in our relationships in bed—but it made his disappearing act all the more devastating. We'd been more vulnerable, more trusting of one another that night than we'd ever been before. So when it became clear that Nick wanted nothing more to do with me, I couldn't help but be relieved I hadn't had sex with him. Because if we'd been having intercourse in our relationship, we would have had it that night for sure. And the idea of doing that with someone who knows in his heart that his heart isn't in it doesn't really sit right with me. My heart was broken as it was. At least I managed to spare it a more fatal blow.

The Nick jokes that started springing up once I'd stopped using a box of tissues a day and started eating human-sized portions again helped me down the road to recovery. "Did you pay the phone bill?" I'd ask Carolyn. "Yeah," she'd reply, "and Nick stopped by today just to say hi." Around my apartment, "when pigs fly" was promptly replaced with "when Nick calls," and socks that never made it back from the laundromat were said to have "pulled a Nick."

I think of him now any time cigarette smoke wafts into my room from an open window in the morning, whenever I hear about alien abductions (he was a nonbe-liever), and whenever I hear any number of songs. I think it's possible you can measure the great loves of your life by how many albums or songs make you think of them. The Lemonheads' *It's a Shame About Ray*, That Petrol Emotion's *Fireproof*, the debut album from a fine Irish band called Engine Alley (Nick loved the band but hated the way the record was produced), The Spindoctors' "Two Princes" and 4 Non Blondes' "What's Up?"—all of them are tied to specific Nick memories that conjure up a different time and what definitely feels like a differ-ent me (and not just because I have less butt and less hair now).

Then there's the whole catalog of songs in the wake of our breakup that Nick would have no clue make me think of him, songs that I would have sent out to him as a Casey Kasem long-distance dedication if I'd thought there was even a remote chance he'd hear, to make it per-fectly clear that I was going on with my life quite happi-ly. That he could *69 his little heart out and never catch me calling just to hear his voice.

Thankfully, the songs that remind me most of him never made it into heavy rotation at the Z100s of the world. I pity the girl who thinks of the man who scorned her whenever she hears Hootie and the Blowfish. Pearl Jam's "Black," however, a song Nick always said made *him* think of *me*, though I never really knew why, has had a pretty long radio life. To this day I listen hard to the lyrics, looking for clues, because I just don't get it.

I also didn't get (rather *couldn't* get) permission from Pearl Jam to reprint those puzzling lyrics for you, so you'll have to listen hard some day for yourself. But the bit I find so baffling is when Eddie Vedder imagines that some day this woman he's singing about will have a great relationship with somebody who isn't him. This fact seems to be causing him a good deal of grief if the plaintive wailing vibe is any indication, because presumably this other guy's going to have this brilliant life and the singer wants to know (and I quote briefly because I can), *"Why can't it be mine?"*

Well, duh, I can't help but think to myself.

Because you left me.

cHAPTER
15

I *find that after any big breakup I face the* prospect of dating—the idea of complete social independence—with great optimism and hope. I envision myself wining and dining with all sorts of fascinating types, none of whom I favor over the others and all of whom find me enthralling. I imagine myself going places I've never gone before and doing things I've never done when I get there—all because some new and exciting man suggested it and I was free to say what the heck. The men involved never make demands, they never grow attached, and they are most definitely not in it for the sex.

This, it took me a number of years to realize, is some sick and twisted idea of mine, some preposterous pipe dream. Not, I repeat, *not* the social practice commonly referred to as "dating."

I'm not sure I've ever known anyone who has ever "dated" successfully. "Dating," the very word embodying variety and levity—flagrant disregard for the concept of a relationship—is perhaps a thing of the past. You may go on a date with someone these days, and it's even possible to have a second one. But if you actually make it to a third outing (and chances are you won't because one of you will become too close for the other one's comfort and ruin things by then), well, then you're not dating, you're "seeing." And quite possibly "sleeping with."

For someone who is definitely not going to complete the sexual act within the first couple of months, if even then—a swinging single without the swing—dating can be particularly difficult. After being in a committed, pressure-free relationship for over a year, however, it can be almost devastating. *What if he really was the one?* you think. *What if Nine Inch Nails lyrics like "I want to fuck you like an animal" replaced "What's your sign?" while I was busy renting movies in Coupleland? What if every guy I meet for the rest of my life wants me to go to bed with him before we've even shared a home-cooked meal? And what if no one—absolutely no one, not even the most hard-up male on the planet—wants the responsibility?*

In any case, this time around I thought I'd gotten off to a pretty good start with Martin. He was English with a particularly charming accent, and I figured, what better way to seek revenge on an Irishman for ditching me? We'd met at a friend's Christmas party a year earlier and hit it off really well. I'd been otherwise committed with Nick, but this time around we hit it off even better (the hosts had hoped we might) and exchanged phone numbers and a bit of spit at night's end.

The following week Martin called to say friends of his from England would be in town on business that weekend, and he invited me to join them for dinner. One of his visitors would be expensing the meal so Martin had suggested going to Boulais. He was joking, obviously, but his friends had actually gone for it.

"Isn't that brilliant?!" he enthused.

Now, if you're anything like me you have absolutely no idea what Boulais is. So you wouldn't have any idea why suggesting having dinner there might be considered a joke, and you'd be at least a little bit apprehensive about what to wear. Perhaps, if you were enterprising like me, you'd turn to your *Zagat* restaurant survey or a New York guide of some variation and discover that Boulais is actually spelled *Bouley* and was perhaps the finest restaurant in all of the Big Apple. Then you'd look through your wardrobe—which doesn't really deserve the title "wardrobe" since it's such a mismatched conglomeration of items of clothing, some of which are old enough to be others' parents—and you'd make damn sure that the one outfit that might be appropriate makes it to the dry cleaners and back in time. Then you'd take a deep breath, plop down on your hand-me-down couch, and let a smile creep over your face. This is it, you'd think. You're really doing it.

Dating.

Going places you've never been before.

Places you can't even spell.

And goddammit you're enjoying it.

Thank god he dumped me, you might even say aloud, or you'd still be that imbecile who had no idea what Bouley was.

Bouley, it turns out, is an absolutely beautiful place with astonishing food. No surprise there. The second you walk in the door (at least in winter), you're bombarded with the sights and smells of an orchard and the dining room exudes an understated elegance. Everyone around you seems to have a refined accent of some sort or another and the Champagne at the bar (because a simple G&T won't do) is on the house if your table's not ready.

Ours wasn't, so we sat in the small bar area with our tall, skinny glasses, smoking Silk Cuts until the rest of our party arrived. Once we were seated, it would be a solid three hours before we moved again. Everyone else opted for the six-course prix fixe meal, which came in at around $75 a plate, so I went with the flow. Eating a ridiculously decadent meal that wasn't costing me a cent definitely qualified as something I'd never done before so I was pretty content. I was sampling *pâté de foie gras*, though I'm not sure I would have if I'd known that it's made from the liver of force-fed geese, and if you took Martin's word for it, I'd never been more charming in my life. I was so witty, insightful, intelligent, and generally persuasive that at night's end, he actually complimented me on being such a good dinner companion, a good "date." I'd found, during my time abroad, that the English and Irish react with at least a little bit of surprise or condescension when faced with an American who understands the meaning of irony and can use it in a sentence, and Martin was no exception. Looking back I'm surprised he didn't pat me on the butt before sending me on my way.

Our next date was a bit less extravagant: dinner and a movie with the friends who'd had the Christmas party and a few other people I didn't know. Still, Martin insisted on paying for everything, and I suppose if he hadn't insisted, *I* would have; he made about four times as much money as I did at the time. After we'd split with the group—mostly married and engaged people, if I recall—Martin and I ducked into Chumleys for a pint, where I confessed my meager salary and challenged him on points like whether or not he really *needed* a cleaning lady.

I was completely nasty to him, actually. On more than one occasion. And I can't say I'm particularly crushed I didn't see him at that fateful Christmas party this year. The verbal abuse was bad enough (though he could certainly give as good as he got), but then I went and slapped him one night. Hard. For no real reason.

When all was said and done, Martin and I had only really fooled around once but it had gotten pretty intense. As he went to take off his own boxers, because I'd no intention of doing so, he heaved, "I want to be inside you," and I was completely turned off. I'm not sure why it even came to this, and looking back he and I would have been much better off as friends. He wasn't really my type physically, so I can only guess that I was lonely, needy, and flattered. I suppose I was looking for someone to take Nick's place and Martin simply wasn't it. We just didn't click on an emotional level and, silly as it sounds, I probably blamed him for that. It really bothered me that he had so much more money to throw around and that he'd say "I want to be inside you" and not mean it figuratively. But what probably bothered me more than anything was the simple fact that he wasn't Nick. I was in desperate need of true affection, and Martin would have been just as happy with a blow-up doll with a couple of snappy comebacks. Or so it seemed to me at the time.

The poor guy. I still feel bad for him.

He had no idea what he was getting himself into.

As far as what *I* was getting myself into—the harsh realities of the singles scene—it was only beginning to come back to me. Suddenly daytime talk shows, which had once been pretty entertaining, inspired fear in me.

Who *are* these people? I used to ask, nestled on a couch in the comfort of coupledom. What's *wrong* with them, I'd wonder, confident in my belief that having sex for money is not an acceptable way to fund your Christmas shopping. Faced again with the prospect of actually having to find my future mate among the vast unknown public, I found myself watching and wondering what was wrong with *me.*

Why do I still have student loans to pay off when there are people putting themselves through college by prostituting? Why am I struggling to make ends meet when it seems everybody and anybody can make a good living as an exotic dancer? How come Jenny Jones' producers haven't called to tell me someone wants to confess a secret crush on me? And perhaps most importantly, could I pick up a guy in thirty seconds at Ricki Lake's on-stage "bar" if I had to?

If my experience with the Fountain Bar is any indication, I'd have a pretty good shot. My roommates and I go there pretty often though, so I guess I've had the benefit of familiarity in that situation. We've been told it's a bit too far away to really qualify as a "local," but the bar that deserves that title—a mere three blocks away—is rumored to be a mob hangout. The Fountain Bar, with its pool table and constant flow of relatively hip young people, is well worth the walk.

Right around the time of Martin's rise and fall I'd picked up pool again. I learned to play as a kid when one of my only real next-door neighbors on the dead-end street where we lived was a guy with Down's syndrome, a veritable shark, with a pool table in his basement. I'd played a bit in college some years later, but foosball was really my game of choice at Harvard. In any case, with my weekends no longer dedicated to Nick, I had more leisure time on my hands and took up the game with renewed vigor. This meant going to places like the Fountain Bar—it's cheaper than going a pool hall—and spending a lot of time in the company of men, who, for whatever reason, tend to play pool with more frequency and therefore skill than women.

A woman who can play pool—one who sinks balls more often than asking whether she's stripes or solids—is a real turn-on for guys, apparently. You could have an oozing third eye on your forehead and a hairy tail sticking out from under your skirt . . . so long as they help your bank shots, not a problem. And so, with my fairly consistent playing, I found myself attracting the eyes of a number of guys who were looking for a little bit more than a pool partner and a good bit more than I was willing to give.

There's really no point in coming up with a fake name for each of the men involved and going into great detail; they had more impact on me taken as a group than any did on his own. There was a guy who was looking for someone to share everything with (some things more quickly than others), who was frustrated by my hesitance to commit or to fool around; a guy who admitted it was just as well I wasn't interested in pursuing anything with him because he wouldn't be able to handle either not having sex or being my first; and a man (a doctor!) who told me he was surprised by my apparent lack of self-esteem before telling me I had a nice ass and asking me to spend the night at his place.

Ah, yes, it was all coming back to me now. Like the time a friend of a friend I went out with a few times begged and pleaded with me to let him spend the night after we'd done nothing more than kiss. I told him I'd really prefer it if he went home—it was late, I had a lot to do the next day, and I was starting to get creeped out by him anyway—so he came up with his idea of a compromise: "I'll stay, but I'll keep my pants on."

Chivalry, I had decided at that moment, was most definitely dead.

I often fantasize about what it would be like if men today had to fight for the woman of their choosing the way they did in legends. Not in duels—to the death—or anything crazy like that. Maybe just in a boxing ring . . .

"In one corner, weighing in at 175 pounds, defending his title as the fastest lay in North America, Martin 'I Want To Be Inside You' Sidwell! . . ."

(*Boos and hisses from the crowd.*)

"And in the other corner, weighing in at 179, two-time winner of the Two-Timing Award, Joseph 'I'll Keep My Pants On' Kahn . . ."

The network commentator cuts in: "Be sure to tune in

next week as Chris 'Are You On the Pill?' Lowe takes on Mike 'I Know You Want to Fuck Me' Sweeney at 8 P.M. Eastern Standard Time. Our coverage begins at 7:30."

Ah, yes, Mike. I almost forgot about him. Lord knows I've tried.

We met in a club and shared a few beers and a few dances before he came to the conclusion that I wanted to fuck him. He actually said it, "I know you want to fuck me," as I tried to tell him politely that I'd like to go home—alone. "If it doesn't happen tonight," he insisted, "it'll happen next time or the time after that." The guy obviously had no idea whom he was dealing with.

If you believe in such a thing as leading someone on, I suppose I'd be found guilty. I've just never bought into the idea that expressing an interest in someone, talking and flirting with them—even kissing them!—should rightfully be taken as a promise of actual sex. Expressing an interest in someone and admitting a certain level of attraction doesn't necessarily mean you want to screw them; it's more likely to mean that you want more information before making that call.

I sometimes think we could avoid a lot of confusion if people wore some kind of sign of intent when they were out socializing, if there were some kind of color coding like in *The Handmaid's Tale*. People looking for sex in red, people looking for a relationship in blue, and people who would be happy with either option in green.

Of course, three colors wouldn't even begin to cover it. The spectrum of opinions on sex and relationships runs through ROYGBIV and everything in between. But when I see people on talk shows going on about how great sleeping around is, how it's nobody's business but their own if they're having safe sex, and how it pays for all their new clothes, I can't help but wonder whether they're really happy. And whether they would be if they got their act together instead of simply "getting theirs." We all know it's not my place, or apparently anybody's, to say.

For a long time I think I thought it was my place. I think I truly believed I could change the men who were desperate to get in my pants, make them better people, by showing them how much more there is to share with a person—physically and emotionally—before sharing sperm. If I gave them everything else they wanted in a relationship, if I was pretty enough, thin enough, smart enough, fun enough . . . . they'd see that intercourse isn't the be-all and end-all. That sharing it—and life—with someone you really love is what matters. That I am worth the wait.

As I drifted through the dating scene this time around, with sex again foremost in the minds of men I met along the way, I finally realized that I already *knew* I was worth the wait, that I had a hell of a lot more to offer than a vagina. It took me years, but I no longer needed every man who expressed an interest in me to confirm it. More important, I woke up to the fact that none of this was worth the effort, that I shouldn't have to do cartwheels to convince someone that it was my right to wait. That I shouldn't have to bend over backwards to prove that I'm not insane for not wanting to have intercourse with every guy who asks me to dinner. That I'm allowed to think that a man who can't conceive of waiting even a month to have sex in a relationship is pathetic and leave it at that. Every time I was out there dating I was worried about convincing guys that I was worth waiting for when I should have been asking myself whether *they* were. Having taken years to pose the question, it took a mere second for me to answer it with a word I knew well.

No.

My grandparents have been married for over fifty years and I'm pretty sure Grandpa didn't ask Grandma if she was on the pill when they kissed for the first time. I'd also be pretty confident in saying that Grandma wasn't looking to get money for a pair of leather boots she'd been eyeing out of the deal.

Yeah, yeah, I know. It's a different world now. Times change. But I'm not sure human nature changes so much. And though nobody but Oprah wants to say it since it sounds so dreadfully uncool, love is still a lot more important than lovin' in the long run. We all get old eventually, and (horror of horrors) we stop having sex. And I know for damn sure that when I'm eightysomething (now there's a television drama idea if I've ever heard one) and me and my crinkly husband are lounging around in our retirement community telling the grandkids about our first date, the words "I know you want to fuck me" won't enter into the picture.

Of course, I might say that to my dear old hubby later that evening, as we go to bed in our separate rooms because, after fifty years, I've decided I don't want to put up with his snoring anymore. But that's another issue altogether.

We'd both know he wouldn't be able to if he tried.

cHAPTER
16

Everyone has a hepatitis story, and if you don't you're about to.

Maybe it's that their cousin's friend had it and was out of work for three months. Or that a friend of theirs had it and wasn't able to drink for a solid year. Or that someone they knew was misdiagnosed with it only to find out they were suffering from liver failure just barely in time to get a life-saving transplant.

My hepatitis story starts on a Friday—February 9, 1996, to be exact.

I'm out with some friends—my college roommates are in town—and I'm not feeling well. I split from the group, deciding it'd be best if I went to sleep, and throw up my dinner the second I get out of my cab, burying recycled *Chicken Francese* in the snow. Over the next couple of days,

I puke until I can't puke any more and decide to go to the clinic.

A doctor wearing knee-high boots tells me I have some kind of stomach bug. Yes, five days is a bit too long to be completely without food, but not to worry. Take these nausea suppressants, start eating, and you'll be fine. Two days later, I call the doctor to tell her I still haven't advanced beyond minimal amounts of applesauce but she merely tells me to plug away.

A few *more* days later, a week and a half after the initial upchuck, I'm sitting in the waiting room at the E.R. watching *General Hospital* and I'm yellow. My eyes are yellow (think Michael Jackson's "Thriller" video), my skin is yellow, and my pee is the color of strong tea. Nurses and doctors take one look at me, know that I have hepatitis, and order the bloodwork to prove it. It's explained to me that I probably have hepatitis A and that I probably got it because someone didn't wash their hands before preparing my food in a restaurant. A particularly unglamorous sickness, it's carried in "fecal matter," which we all know is just a nice way of saying shit. Hepatitis B, I'm informed, is a more serious strain which is sexually transmitted and can only be ruled out by follow-up bloodwork. The doctor says he's going to give me an IV to get some fluids into my rapidly dehydrating body before sending me home to ride it out, and asks me whether there's anyone waiting for me. I tell him my boyfriend is and he asks whether it's okay if he tells him what's going on. I assure him that I've nothing to hide and give him his name.

My boyfriend arrives at my side, holds my hand while fluids drip through the IV, and escorts me home, where I'm to drink lots of liquids and get lots of rest. He transforms himself into Supernurse, keeping my Brita filter full and cooking me flavorless meals against his better culinary instincts when I begin to feel up to it. My brother drives me out to my dad's place where I can recuperate with the benefit of peace, quiet, and cable TV.

A week later my boyfriend has, according to his doctor, a stomach bug, but I know better. A week after that he's yellow and bored and I'm the one playing nurse. I become a regular at the video store, make him a variety of Jell-O's, and take his temperature three or four times a day. Together, we've created an alternate reality— Hepatitis World—and I wonder whether it will ever show up on an episode of *Sliders*. The adventurers through alternate worlds will travel to a world where people are either yellow, emaciated, exhausted, bored and feeling sorry for themselves, or tending to someone who is while trying to maintain their own sanity. Marriage vows don't include the "in sickness and in health" bit because, in Hepatitis World, that'd be like saying "in spring and fall."

Back in this world, both myself and my loved one finally recovered, I mentally tick off the familiar vows:

"For better, for worse . . ."

Yeah, I'd say we covered that when he had rats in his kitchen and had to move in with me for two months.

"For richer, for poorer . . ."

Yup, been there. Or hope to very soon.

"In sickness and in health . . . "

Got that covered.

So far, so good, I think, but the "'til death do us part" bit's the biggie, after all.

Mark Waeldner is one of the most amazing men I have ever met and I'm not just saying that because he thought I was beautiful even when I was yellow. He is intelligent, insightful, kind, and admirably secure in who he is, and if he has a jealous bone in his body it's certainly not one he drags off into a corner and chews on for hours. He's the only man I've ever met who, like me, hates made-for-television movies but cries anyway if he gets sucked into an emotional one, and will actually buy your horoscope out of curiosity to test your compatibility. His devotion to the people in his life—a passionate, sometimes irrational devotion—is matched only by his devotion to the UMass basketball team, which I was eternally grateful consists solely of men. I don't think I could have handled the competition.

Of course, I didn't know any of this when I first met Mark and I didn't want to. I was in love with Nick at the time and no one—especially not an environmental engineer who, it was rumored, had little graduation cap icons and stuff on his résumé—was going to ruin that for me.

Still, Mark did his best. Not that he's a homewrecker or anything like that. At first he didn't even know I had a boyfriend. It's just that we clicked immediately—and Mark didn't see any point in denying that, not until I gave him a reason to. Once I told him about Nick, he was perfectly willing to be my friend—whatever I wanted that to mean—and for a while that's how things went. But the seed of romance had been planted, and with it the seed of doubt about me and Nick. Actually, that seed was already growing. Mark . . . well, let's just say he watered it.

The first time I met him, he'd come to visit my roommate and friend Cathleen (remember the rebel nerd?), one of his best friends from college. I remember the first time he walked into my apartment as if it was yesterday. I was looking for something in a desk drawer, maybe a pen, and, seeing motion out of the corner of my eye, looked up for a second. Our eyes met, but I was already on my way to looking away and had no choice but to pull a classic daytime soap–quality double take—one that a cunning director would no doubt use again in a slow motion playback during a later episode when Mark and Tara, after many a struggle (perhaps one "dies" and comes back to life), finally walk down the aisle. Mark was carrying a case of beer, and swears to this day it was the Molson that caught my eye. In that instant, I had an overwhelming sense of already knowing him.

We *had* actually met once before, but just barely. A few years earlier, I'd gone to visit Cathleen at UMass and since it was raining, she'd coerced Mark into driving her to the bus stop to pick me up before he left town for the weekend. Basically I'd climbed into the backseat of his car, said thanks for the ride, and climbed out. We'd hardly paid attention to each other and I'm not even convinced I saw his face. So much for love at first sight.

This time around, as a group of seven or eight people headed to a restaurant in my neighborhood, Mark and I ended up walking and talking side by side, and I'll confess—with no disrespect to Nick—that I made a point of sitting near him at our long table. I wasn't plotting or even considering an infidelity, just taking a healthy interest in a friend of a friend. One who happened to be a guy. Or at least that's the way we rationalize it—those of us who are in relationships and thrive, just once in a while, on the attention of another member of the opposite sex, a significant interest on the part of someone who isn't your significant other. It's called flirting, it's supposed to be harmless, and in most cases it is. Usually it only takes a little while before the novelty wears off, and when it does you want nothing more than to go straight home and call your steady.

That realization was a bit long in coming for me and it pissed me off to no end. I was mad that I was being tempted. Mad that I'd slow-danced with Mark, never really having done that with Nick, and really mad that I'd enjoyed it. Today I'm just mad that I don't remember what song it was. Mark always said he thought it was "Hotel California," the only problem being that I wouldn't have danced to that song if someone had threatened to tar and feather me.

When Mark came to visit another time, a night out with a group culminated in a one-on-one conversation in my kitchen that lasted until about five in the morning, Mark and I talking about Nick and me and how things were really going, which by this time was not well. I was committed to working things out, however, and Mark was prepared to bow out gracefully. The two of them would eventually meet, though Nick didn't really pay much attention to Mark, having no real reason to, at least not one he was aware of. Some months later, after Mark had moved to Sweden where he was finishing the research toward his master's degree, he wrote me a letter telling me he was glad he got the chance to meet Nick and see what a good guy he was, a guy who seemed to deserve me.

Of course, that letter arrived a few days after Nick had dropped his I'm-not-sure-I-want-the-pressure bomb and I wasn't so convinced he deserved me after all. I wrote back, instinctively spilling my guts about why Nick and I were better off apart, and asked Mark to show me that letter if I ever got back together with Nick. He still has it; mind you, I'm pretty sure I won't ever need to read it again.

It was the start of a ten-month correspondence, during which Mark and I went from being friends (acquaintances, really) to lovers, though you may have a hard time understanding how such a thing could happen through the mail and I'm not sure we understood it ourselves. We saw each other only once during those ten months, when Mark came home for the holidays, and having established that there was still a strong connection and very strong attraction between us, we began to send letters with even more passion and frequency. Sometimes I'd get three in a week.

Then there was the not-so-small matter of the phone bill. Luckily for me it was *Mark's* phone bill. Since you don't get itemized bills in Sweden, we could only guess that our longest conversation—close to three hours— cost him over $200. The biggest one that ever appeared on my bill was a measly $32. He'd call me from Gothenburg, then when he was traveling around Europe a call from Manchester, another from Glastonbury, St. Ives, all in the lead-up to a romantic rendezvous/reunion we'd planned in Dublin. I was making my first return visit to Ireland—I'd been home for almost two years already—and Mark was going to be there at the same time.

I suggested we meet in a pub but he insisted it be out-doors. I warned him; it was Ireland, it would probably rain. He said it wouldn't. Pubs weren't incredibly roman-tic. I had to do better. So I suggested the gates of Trinity University and Mark agreed.

Friday, July 21, 1995. 7 o'clock. Trinity. The date was set.

I was so nervous I thought I'd throw up and as I set out toward Trinity, having already spent a week in Ireland revisiting old haunts, it started raining. *I told you so*, I thought to myself, as I quickened my pace to avoid the drops only to slow it again in fear of arriving on the scene first. I swear the second I set foot on the cobblestone path leading up to Trinity's main courtyard the sun broke through again. I saw a figure looming in the distance, a red rose in hand, and since I'd never seen Mark with any facial hair I wasn't sure it was him. I'd gotten a pretty drastic haircut since I'd last seen him and we were between five and ten feet apart before he actually looked up and recognized me. The embrace that followed was long and passionate and I feel like I know every detail of it today.

And not only because I have about twenty-four pictures of it.

See, Mark had been traveling through the UK with Andy, an English guy whose long, yellow-blonde hair makes him look more like a Viking than anything, and Andy was pretty handy with his camera. I'd never met him before, but he'd been shown a picture of me and was staked out at Trinity. He shot an entire roll of film, sometimes taking pictures from a mere ten feet away while I remained completely oblivious to his presence. Mark even said, "You want to say hi to Andy?" to me at one point, but it didn't really register.

Upon our return to the States, I framed three of those pictures, pictures that ooze romance and drama, and hung them over my bed, a bed I began to share with Mark on a regular basis when he moved to New York and started his new job. We continued our written correspondence in a black-and-white marble notebook passed back and forth between us, but reveled in each other's physical presence. Quite quickly, we became what you'd call an established couple and the love between us grew stronger.

This isn't to say there weren't problems, even early on. It's just that we had learned so much about each other and seen such good in the way we could communicate through our letters that we saw problems as bumps in the road, obstacles to be overcome for the sake of a greater cause, a greater love. There was something challenging about it, and something very "adult," for lack of a better word. It was as if every day we were discovering something new about ourselves and one other, not the least of which was that when it came to romantic histories, we might as well have been from different planets.

Mark could count the "dates" he'd been on on his fingers, while I'd need an abacus. He'd had three relationships that lasted longer than a year and a half while I average approximately 4.8 months. He'd had sex with each of his girlfriends before me and me with none of my boyfriends before him. These issues weren't very easily brushed aside, though I believe we were able to come to a workable understanding with time.

From where Mark stood, there was the issue of the numbers. I've been intimate with a lot more people than Mark had and picturing me with them didn't particularly thrill him. The way he saw it, he was in love, or at least thought he was, with all of the women he'd had sex with and he simply couldn't fathom how I could be intimate with so many guys I barely knew.

For my part, the idea of Mark's having had sex with other women—women who were still friends of his and whom he hoped I'd someday meet—bothered me; I couldn't help it. I've held on to my virginity—admittedly by a thread—because I want to have it to share with the man I decide to share the rest of my life with. The fact that Mark has already shared the one act I value most with other women made me wonder whether I'd wasted my time. This was not new to me. I guess since for a long time I imagined my soulmate of sorts out there somewhere, waiting to find me, waiting *for* me, the idea that I could end up with someone whose first has been relegated to a picture in their high school yearbook has always been disheartening. On an emotional level, something about it just feels wrong.

Still, I really did understand how Mark could have his own difficulties accepting my sexual past and was forced to really examine my own behavior closely for the first time ever. I've always felt that on some level the fact I've never given all I have to give makes up for the flings. But as I studied my own history so that I could explain it to Mark, I found that I wasn't so thrilled with it either; the fact that I hadn't made the mistake of having actual sex when I wasn't ready didn't mean that I hadn't made other mistakes. A lot of them. Looking back on it all, it seemed there was a certain desperation driving me—this need to find a man to make my life whole—and I allowed it to take me places and let me do things I would no longer feel comfortable doing. It took loving and being loved by someone who wanted to understand that behavior, that desperation, to help me finally come to terms with it. And, once confronted by someone who understood my ideals but challenged whether I'd really lived up to them, I was able to come full circle and realize that I don't want to be doing any of it with just anybody—whether it's intercourse or not. That was the original idea, after all.

I no longer feel that need to find "the one" with such urgency, in no small part due to the way in which Mark and I eventually brought our year-plus romantic involvement to an end. More than anything it was sad. Not necessarily devastating or horrific and hardly as dramatic as any number of other breakups in my life. It was just really, really *sad*—that two people who are just now really starting to understand what they want out of life found that their visions didn't overlap enough for their own good in spite of the love they shared. Ending things before we hurt each other anymore, before the frustration of not understanding one another on some fundamental levels destroyed the chance for friendship, just seemed like the right thing to do. Some friends and family didn't understand; they thought it was simply Mark's being a little bit country (enjoys backpacking and the like) and my being a little bit rock 'n' roll that caused the trouble and that that was surely surmountable; but Mark and I knew it ran deeper than that.

Deciding that we would be better off as friends felt like the first completely mature decision I'd ever made in my love life to date. And having come to that level of maturity, having come to understand that I know what I want and still believe it's out there, I don't think there's any going back. After having the relationship I had with Mark, I simply can't see myself hooking up with random men or even fooling around with a guy I've only gone on a few dates with. It's not who I want to be. Even if it *was* who I want to be (though I'm not sure why anyone would strive for such a thing), I'm not sure I *could* be it. My sober hepatitis period put alcohol in its place in my life, and it's a much smaller one now, far away from the bedroom.

I sometimes wonder whether there's something wrong with me that I haven't found the right person yet. There's a lot of pressure in society—and certainly in my extended family—to pair off and reproduce. But I have to remind myself that I'm hardly the last single person in the world. I'm not even the last—or necessarily the oldest—"virgin."

Maybe Mark and I could have made it. Maybe it's the curse of our generation that we make things more complicated than they really are. Maybe they really are more complicated and we're the only ones smart enough to realize it. Maybe it's simply that we weren't ready to settle down. Or settle.

Oddly enough, I do feel ready for the responsibility of sex now, and there were times when I thought very hard about doing it with Mark. He was an incredible, caring lover and I have no doubt it would have been a good experience. But I was intellectualizing the decision, challenging myself to think of a good reason not to do it with such a wonderful man, when the truth is I know I'll feel it in my heart when it's right.

There was absolutely no pressure from Mark to go ahead with it; I'm not sure we would have lasted as long if that hadn't been the case. Still, I asked him pretty often whether it bothered him that we weren't having sex and he always said, no absolutely not. And it wasn't just because he was getting his kicks anyway; unlike people who think it's all the same, Mark believed there was a difference between what we were doing and making love. He didn't see that as a bad thing—that he was being denied a certain kind of intimacy he wanted or deserved—but saw it, I think, as something to look forward to. "Sex isn't necessarily the best way to show someone you love them," he wrote to me once. And in the end, I guess we realized that going out with them wasn't either.

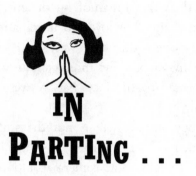

IN
PARTING . . .

This is a happy ending. *I feel like I have to tell you* that right out because it's not the kind of hit-you-over-the-head, cue triumphant music, fade to black, roll credits happy ending you may be used to.

In the Hollywood happy ending, I'd probably be engaged to be married and would have tried on my mother's white wedding dress to find it's a perfect fit. Then I'd walk down the aisle, do the I do's and fly Virgin Atlantic Airlines to the Virgin Islands where, secure in my husband's love for me and mine for him, I'd make love to him with everything—and every body part—I've got. In the morning, I'd order a Virgin Mary with my breakfast in bed just to see how it feels to say the word and not be one.

Or maybe it'd go something like this: I'd somehow get cast in a "You're Worth Waiting For" public service television spot only to receive floods of letters, one of which ends up being from the virginal man of my dreams. We'd have dinner and, overwhelmed by love and anticipation of things to come, we'd elope within mere weeks of meeting one another before living happily, monogamously ever after, our hearts warmed by the fact that we were each other's "one and only."

In truth, the happy ending here is not the stuff of great cinematic moments. There's not really a whole lot of action involved so the lights and camera would pretty much be a waste. In the end there's simply acceptance—of who I am and what I want out of life and sex. This may not be very exciting for you, and I apologize if that's the case, but for me it has made a world of difference.

Now, when friends say that my not having intercourse but doing pretty much everything else is akin to arbitrarily deciding to eat every flavor of ice cream except chocolate chip, I only contemplate the argument for a minute before putting the matter aside and getting on with my life; there was a time not so long ago when such an "accusation" would have had me ruminating on the nature of chocolate chip ice cream for weeks.

More importantly, the embarrassment factor—such a huge part of the virgin experience—is gone. I mean, if there's anything people should be embarrassed about it's things like marrying your daughter's ex-husband, making a fool of yourself on college *Jeopardy!* (don't they all), or being stupid enough to have unprotected sex. At this point, if it got out that I'm a sucker for *Doogie Howser* reruns or have an inexplicable fondness for cows, one that actually impelled me to spend hard-earned cash on a rosy-cheeked stuffed one on a ski trip to Vermont last winter, I'd be much more upset.

The point is that I don't really care what anybody thinks anymore—about my virginity, Doogie, anything. I know that for me, the right time, place, guy, and circumstances have yet to coincide. Me and my standards being what we are, it may not happen for some time, but I'm hardly going to isolate myself from the world or even lie to it anymore. You know the deal, two paths diverged, I took the one less traveled and that is where it got me. So be it.

The fact that my Catholic upbringing got me started down that path early on doesn't really bother me. It's not that I've never questioned things I've been taught; I just haven't felt the need to reject all of them. We're all products of our environment, our families, and most importantly, our experiences as individuals moving through the world. Having imagined where I'd be today if I'd misused intercourse as often as I misused other forms of intimacy, I can't say I feel the need to rebel against my own sense of what's right for me and what isn't. I'm not sure where that sense comes from, and I never will be, but I've grown to trust it—and even wish I'd paid a little more attention to it at times. And over the years, I've learned that I can't change it any more than I can my favorite color or the fact that I could never live happily as a vegetarian. I love green and I love red meat. (Green meat, I can do without.)

A character in John B. Keane's *Letters of a Love-Hungry Farmer* suggests to his virginal friends, "A good screw would leave all your philosophy in the shade," and there are times when I still wonder whether he's right. It's possible that when all is said and done and the lucky guy has fallen asleep beside me, I'll lie there and say to myself, "You idiot, you could have been doing that for years!" It's also possible I'll think, "That's it? *That* was what I was waiting for?!" But I don't have any romanticized notions of the mechanics of sex, and unlike *90210*'s Andrea, I'm not going to be studying myself in the mirror the following morning and asking friends if I look different. And, in spite of an ever-increasing desire for what I imagine intercourse feels like, I'm not expecting a mind-blowing orgasm or the best sexual experience of my life. The physical pleasure of it isn't nearly so important to me as the emotional release of giving myself to someone—the right one— body and soul.

Because I want that truly unique experience in my life, because that combination of spiritual and physical connection is something I believe in, I sometimes wonder whether it's inevitable I'll end up with a man who hasn't really experienced that before either. Not that he'll necessarily be a virgin (and with men, there's never really the question of whether he is or isn't, is there?), but I think it's possible he'll be someone who simply never really got it quite right before me. And wants to.

For a long time I was looking for someone who I thought was worthy, someone who understood and who deserved a gift of this magnitude—the ultimate gift that keeps on giving. But, having done many a thing because it seemed like a good idea at the time myself, that feeling of superiority has been replaced gradually over the years with a quieter feeling of empowerment and pride at having stuck to my guns.

I know, simply, that in the end it will be with someone who loves me and whom I love back—unconditionally. I also know that when I do have sex and do so for all the right reasons, it will be the biggest gift I've ever given anyone in my life. I just can't believe how long it took me to understand that I'd be giving it to myself. I'm supposed to be one of the bright ones.

I honestly can't say whether it'll be my wedding gift to myself. Though I like the idea of waiting until I'm married, I don't know whether I'll hang on until vows have been exchanged or simply until it feels like the right thing to do. These are things I'll have to feel out along the way. But the one thing I'm sure of—and I can't say this would have been true even six months ago—is that I'm ready for it, and when the right times comes I'll know it.

For that matter you probably will, too.

The earth may very well grind to a halt.